Research in Medicine
Planning a project – writing a thesis

Third Edition

D0756196

Research in Medicine

Planning a project – writing a thesis

Third Edition

Juliet Usher-Smith, MB, BChir, PhD (Cantab)
Murray Edwards College,
University of Cambridge, Cambridge, UK

George Murrell, MBBS (Adelaide), DPhil (Oxon), MD (UNSW)
Department of Orthopaedic Surgery,
University of New South Wales,
St. George Hospital Campus, Sydney, Australia

Harold Ellis, CBE, FRCS, MCh, DM (Oxon)
Department of Anatomy,
Guy's Hospital Campus, London, UK

Christopher Huang, ScD (Cantab), DM (Oxon)
Physiological Laboratory,
Department of Biochemistry,
and Murray Edwards College,
University of Cambridge, Cambridge, UK

With line drawings by
David Langdon, OBE, FRSA

CAMBRIDGE
UNIVERSITY PRESS

CAMBRIDGE UNIVERSITY PRESS
Cambridge, New York, Melbourne, Madrid, Cape Town, Singapore,
São Paulo, Delhi, Dubai, Tokyo

Cambridge University Press
The Edinburgh Building, Cambridge CB2 8RU, UK

Published in the United States of America by Cambridge University Press, New York

www.cambridge.org
Information on this title: www.cambridge.org/9780521132282

First published 2010

Printed in the United Kingdom at the University Press, Cambridge

A catalogue record for this publication is available from the British Library

Library of Congress Cataloguing in Publication Data
Research in medicine: planning a project, writing a thesis. –3rd ed. /
   Juliet Usher-Smith ... [et al.]; with line drawings by David Langdon.
      p. ; cm.
   Rev. ed. of: Research in medicine / George Murrell, Christopher Huang,
   Harold Ellis. 2nd ed. 1999.
   Includes bibliographical references and index.
   ISBN 978-0-521-13228-2 (pbk.)
   1. Medicine–Research.   2. Medical writing.   3. Dissertations, Academic.
   I. Usher-Smith, Juliet A.   II. Murrell, George, 1960- Research in medicine.
   [DNLM: 1. Dissertations, Academic as Topic.   2. Education, Medical,
   Graduate.   3. Biomedical Research.   4. Writing. W 20 R432 2010]
   R852.M87 2010
    610.72–dc22   2009050379

ISBN 978-0-521-13228-2 Paperback

Contents

Preface

Looking back on my own scientific work I should say that it shows no great originality but a certain amount of business instinct which leads to the selection of a profitable line. (E. D. Adrian, autobiographical notes [A. L. Hodgkin (1979): *Biographical Memoirs of Fellows of the Royal Society* 25, 1–73.])

Doctors and medical students experience a training directed primarily towards clinical practice. Yet, increasing numbers of the more successful additionally devote time to advancing knowledge, often while working for a research or intercalated Honours degree. Similarly, science students are selected for postgraduate work mainly through university degree results. However, little is said about the qualities one requires for successfully completing a research programme, and the extent to which these differ from what makes a successful doctor or undergraduate student. No doubt one requires originality, creativity or flair, but to attempt to define or expand upon these would be beyond the direct scope of this short book. Additionally, modern medicine encompasses an enormous breadth of subjects, and research is among the most individual of endeavours.

Nevertheless, one can discuss some of the more practical problems associated with pursuing research and working for a thesis and a capacity to tackle these fulfils a necessary, even if not a sufficient, condition for a successful research programme. We hope we have commented helpfully upon at least some of these hurdles, even if only briefly in a general way. If we thereby provoke constructive thought, even if not agreement, we shall feel we have achieved our object and have offered assistance to those seeking masterships, doctorates and honours degrees.

We are grateful to Cambridge University Press for encouraging us to write this third edition, particularly in view of the current resurgence of interest in clinical and translational medical research, and in the training and career development of future physician-scientists who will carry this out. These, and other developments that include current alterations in the structure of undergraduate and postgraduate medical education in the UK, are reflected in this current revision of the text. We have additionally taken the opportunity to refine and bring other information given in many of the sections up to date. In this third edition, we remember our indebtedness to Dr Richard Barling of Cambridge University Press, and Professor Richard Adrian of the Physiological Laboratory, University of Cambridge, for their guidance and encouragement in writing the first edition. Finally, we particularly appreciate David Langdon's humorous and sensitive cartoon illustrations of what might otherwise have been rather over-serious material.

Juliet Usher-Smith
George Murrell
Harold Ellis
Christopher Huang

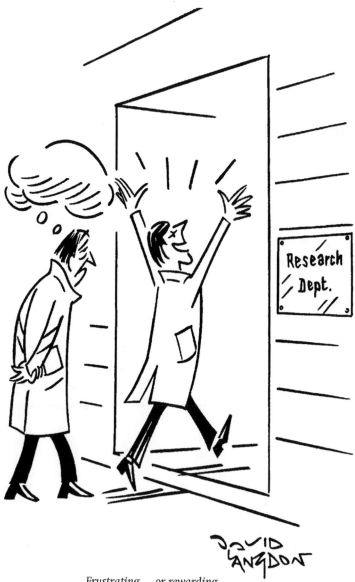

Frustrating ... or rewarding ...

1

Introduction

Aims of this book

This guide was written primarily for medical students and practitioners considering whether to attempt a programme involving original research in the medical and biological sciences. The author who initiated this text (George Murrell) read for a medical degree, did a stint in research and has now returned to clinical medicine (orthopaedic surgery) with an academic interest. He was then joined by two others, one of whom (Christopher Huang) first qualified in medicine and has subsequently remained in research, and another (Harold Ellis) who has had a primarily academic clinical career. In this third edition, they are now joined by Juliet Usher-Smith, who completed a combined MB/PhD programme and is now at the early stages of combining clinical practice with research. Accordingly, the authors themselves represent the major groups and career stages of people who do medical research.

Individuals have different reasons for wishing to do research, which include gaining a higher degree, furthering their medical career or simply taking a break from clinical practice. Such a pursuit can be incredibly exhilarating and rewarding. Alternatively, it can be an endless, lonely, boring and frustrating exercise. The aim of this handbook is to guide the potential medical postgraduate candidate away from the latter predicament. It is not intended to dictate the researcher's own originality, creativity or scientific approach. Rather, it is organized around a sequence of practical steps directed at the more pragmatic questions:

'What steps do I take?'
'When and where do I start?'
'How do I get to the end of the tunnel?'
'What do I do next?'

We thereby hope to alleviate unnecessary anxiety and save the reader valuable time and energy that could then be used in a more productive way. We have accordingly set out much of the text in a simple, didactic format.

Much of what we outline will be simple common sense, but we hope that our presentation will enable the potential researcher to pick out 'the wood from the trees' and assist the reader to his or her task with greater efficiency and confidence. Our comments are directed largely at doctors undertaking clinical or experimental research. However, the basic principles of maintaining an effective individual research programme are also applicable to those pursuing Public Health or Primary Care research and those in purely scientific careers.

It is worth pointing out at this stage that the focus for this book will be on research as opposed to audit. Although the distinctions between the two are often blurred, research involves developing and testing new hypotheses in order to advance our knowledge and understanding of a specific topic, whereas clinical audit is a quality improvement process that aims to improve patient care and outcomes by carrying out a systematic review of current practice against established guidelines and implementing change. Whilst becoming involved in audit can therefore be a useful prelude to research, the process itself is quite different.

Outline

This guide is organized in the chronological order of the steps most doctors take when pursuing a research programme. Everyone first has to decide whether he or she wishes to pursue research and then, if the decision is made to enter research, the decision of when to embark on it must be made. The next stage of choosing a research degree, a supervisor and a project and applying for research positions is perhaps the most critical. After that, all research programmes tend to follow the same pattern. Following the necessary background preparation in the area to be studied, one establishes and develops methods to be used in the research project. Time is then needed to assess the limitations of these methods and to develop one's experimental skills to a level where they yield valid results and overcome the inevitable frustration. There then follows serious hypothesis testing and obtaining and analysing results. Finally, the results are written up and communicated, either through publishing papers or presenting at scientific meetings and, ultimately, in the form of a thesis and/or a *viva voce* examination.

The time and emphasis bearing on each of these steps varies with person, project and research supervisor. In particular, the prominence of the phase of frustration depends largely on the circumstances and the good or ill fortune of the investigator. In addition, the time taken to write up the thesis or research papers varies greatly, tending to increase sharply with the total time set aside by the doctor for research.

Summary
- Research in Medicine is, for the most part, exhilarating and rewarding, but without adequate planning and support it can be an endless, frustrating exercise.
- This book aims to provide practical advice for anyone considering medical research.
- This book is organized in chronological order, from deciding whether to do research through the planning stage to writing a thesis.

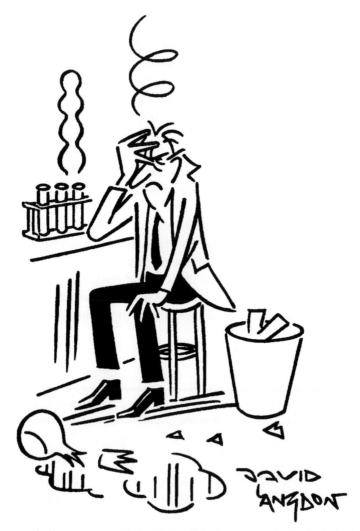

Great potential for disasters . . .

2

Deciding whether to do research

Research experience is increasingly important in today's fight for jobs and so the aspiring clinician may leap, somewhat reluctantly, into a research programme without carefully assessing its processes, outcomes, advantages and disadvantages. Some considerations as to whether or not one should do research at all are presented here.

The challenge

Research by its very nature offers a tremendous intellectual and personal challenge and has the potential to unearth information that may help the wider community.

Becoming a better clinician

A number of desirable qualities are necessary for, and consequently, developed in, research. These include an open, inquiring mind, logical thought, careful analysis of previous research with a mild degree of scepticism, an understanding of the processes necessary to achieve the presented result, self-discipline and self-sufficiency. It can be argued that many of these are also of considerable value in clinical practice. Almost any established clinician who has spent time in research during training, whether they are surgeons in district general hospitals, physicians in private practice or general practitioners, will tell you that they regard themselves better doctors as a result of this experience. They find themselves more able to analyse a clinical problem, appraise the results of their management of patients and assess objectively the latest claims from scientists, colleagues and pharmaceutical companies because of their exposure to the scientific method.

As part of an academic career

Without doubt, research achievement, including a higher degree by thesis, is essential for a career in academic medicine. Most people who decide on a career in university medicine do so from an interest in research and teaching; it is not invariably true, but it is surprising how often the two do go together! It is a hard fact that subsequent promotion in such a career depends on a proven research record with relevant publications in reputable and refereed journals.

Competing in the job market

Selecting one applicant rather than another in appointments for medical jobs has always been a difficult process. The ability to conduct research and publish research papers has become an increasingly important factor, even in non-academic medicine. There are now sections on presentations and publications in all the application forms at all levels and an expectation that all doctors will, at some point in their career, be involved in research. Several good papers in reputable journals consequently serve a candidate well for future employment. However, one must remember that two or three years in an unproductive pursuit of research away from any clinical experience, leading to a few esoteric papers in obscure journals, may not enhance your status with future employers.

Fame

Potential for fame arising from ones' research findings on a small scale is reasonably good. You might find yourself making significant new discoveries, getting a difficult assay to work or solving a theoretical problem. However, to reach great heights requires years of dedication, insight and luck, and there is great potential for disasters (unsuccessful projects, infected cultures, broken glassware and machinery, etc.) and wasting months or years in the pursuit of what seems to be an endless, unsolvable problem.

Lifestyle

If you want continual reassurance and direction, research is not for you. Self-assurance, independent thought and the willingness to take a chance are valuable in research. The working day is structured by you, not your employer, but this does leave greater freedom for other activities. This increased flexibility may be a particular factor for female doctors planning to have a family or wishing to work part-time. However, the distinction between work and rest is less clear and there is great pressure on you to work at home and at weekends. Monetary rewards while in research are also generally less than in clinical medicine.

Summary

- Think carefully before embarking on medical research.
- There are many different reasons for wishing to do research, including to become a better clinician, gain a higher degree, further your medical career or simply take a break from clinical practice.

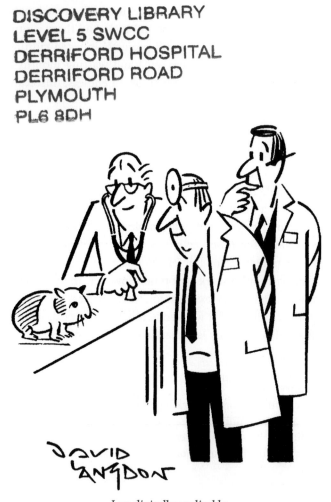

Less clinically applicable...

3

Deciding when to do research

Biological scientists not proceeding to do medicine usually attempt their higher degrees immediately after their first degree, often continuing an interest arising from an honours degree project. Others return to university after a time working in industry. Medical students or doctors have a number of options, each with particular advantages and disadvantages. These relate both to the implications of taking 'time out' for research on future medical career prospects, and to the effects of this timing on the academic quality of the research. The main options for timing of research in medicine are:

1. Prior to medical training.
2. During undergraduate medical training.
3. Between undergraduate medical training and starting clinical work.
4. During clinical training.

Ultimately, the choice of when to do research will depend on a large number of both personal and professional factors and what is 'best' for one person may be very different from what is 'best' for another. Here we consider some of the advantages and disadvantages of the various options. Much of the text here relates to medical students and doctors within the UK, but details of the differences in other countries are included at the end of the chapter.

1. Prior to medical training

Research after a basic science degree may be very helpful for gaining entry to medical school, and often sets the groundwork for each of the later steps.

2. Research during undergraduate medical training

A year or more of research taken during undergraduate training, leading to a BSc, MPhil or PhD, is a well-recognized step in many universities. Indeed, this is often actively encouraged for the more successful students.

A number of medical students become sufficiently interested in basic sciences, or at least particular aspects of them, before they begin the clinical component of their undergraduate course. This is particularly so if they have read for an honours degree, or have included an intercalated BSc as part of their basic medical course, and feel they would like to proceed directly to completing a research degree before their clinical course. Under such circumstances, you have the advantage of having basic scientific concepts fresh in your mind and this can be helpful, at least at the beginning. Doing your research at this stage also avoids disruption to clinical training later. However, your research may be confined to experimental scientific work. You may have neither the knowledge of, nor the access to, a clinical environment or clinical resources, except under very particular circumstances determined by the interests and background of your supervisor. You will also have to complete your work within a strict time limit in order to rejoin your medical course, at the appropriate point in the academic year. Clinical schools are often helpful and understanding to those who wish to take time out before their clinical studies. However, deferral is necessarily for a fixed time, limited by the start of the academic year. It is also more than likely that the area in which you pursue research will have little or no relationship to your eventual interests, as you will not have had opportunities to explore your options in the clinical field at either the undergraduate or postgraduate level.

An increasing number of medical schools, both in the UK and the US, offer their academically most successful students the option, and financial and academic support, to pursue MB-PhD or MD-PhD programmes. These structured programmes combine the undergraduate component of clinical training with a research programme leading to a PhD. This would permit you to obtain a continued clinical exposure through your PhD programme, although the extent to which your research can cover clinical material would be restricted by the fact that you would not yet have secured your full clinical qualifications. In addition, such courses are frequently highly demanding and often restricted to the most successful of the preclinical student intake. The extent to which clinical teaching commitments impinge upon and interfere with the basic research will also vary, depending on the medical school in which you pursue such a programme. Nevertheless, such courses do combine some of the advantages of pursuing research soon after your preclinical course, whilst maintaining exposure to clinical medicine at the same time. They also signal your academic interests or capacity in future job applications, particularly to prospective employers interested in clinicians with an academic interest, for which specific career pathways are developing in conjunction with UK (and US) funding bodies.

3. Research between the primary medical degree and starting clinical work

This next option, which we would *not* recommend, is to do research between the primary medical degree and starting clinical work. This option almost completely prevents a subsequent career in clinical medicine. A year as a Foundation year 1 doctor or an intern is a prerequisite in all countries for practising medicine. To go back to this after time in research is logistically and psychologically difficult. In addition, it is during this first year that you acquire much of your basic knowledge of medical practice, and this could be very beneficial to your subsequent medical research.

4. Research during postgraduate medical training

The decision to do research during your postgraduate medical training requires careful consideration of how you are going to combine this with your clinical work. Ideally, you would take a post which includes a year or more out of clinical practice specifically for research as a part of a planned rotation, or arrange with your employer to return to the clinical training programme after your period of research. Many training programmes allow you to apply for out-of-programme experiences which enable you to take a year or more out of clinical training without losing your training post. Deliberately taking a longer research post without anything definite to go to when this comes to an end can make returning to clinical practice difficult.

To help with this, there are now an increasing number of academic clinical posts developing within the UK which are designed to provide a career structure for doctors wishing to combine research with clinical practice. At present these include:

- Academic Foundation Programmes – for newly qualified doctors where four months of the two-year programme are spent in a specific area of research;
- Academic Clinical Fellowships – three- or four-year programmes for doctors in the early years of speciality training where typically 25% of the time is spent on research to prepare a competitive application for a training fellowship for a higher degree or postdoctoral fellowship; and
- Clinical Lecturer posts – four-year programmes designed for doctors with a PhD/MD or equivalent, who already have specialty training experience, to provide opportunities for post-higher degree research.

Following this career path, you would complete a two-year Foundation Programme and then spend three or four years as an Academic Clinical Fellow acquiring both clinical training in your chosen speciality and basic research skills in order then to apply for funding for a research degree. This has the advantage that you will have the specialist clinical knowledge to select areas that you regard as being interesting and important and will have had time to get to know potential departments and research supervisors. However, a research stint seems a more noticeable interruption of career at this stage and one then also has to consider financial implications and family commitments.

An alternative is to follow a traditional medical training path and then apply for funding for a research degree at a time of your choice, either before or during clinical speciality training. Although you will not have time set aside during your clinical training to plan and prepare a research proposal, this option gives you more independence over the timing of your period of research and additionally gives you the added flexibility to choose to apply for a research degree immediately after completing your Foundation training before starting clinical speciality training. Although at that stage you will not yet have the specialist medical knowledge which comes from working for postgraduate medical examinations, you will have a full medical qualification and so be eligible for, and have access to, clinical projects. Completing a research degree at this early stage can also help when it comes to applying for later speciality training. However, you must also bear in mind that you will have left clinical medicine at a relatively junior stage in your career, and so will have to be prepared to re-enter at the bottom of the medical hierarchy after your 'time out'.

Arrangements in the US and Australia

As in the UK, career paths in Australia or the USA may well change and/or be given different names in the near future. Nevertheless, similar general principles apply concerning the different principal time-points when research could be undertaken. In the USA, many aspiring doctors do some research during their undergraduate degree, which helps them get into medical school in the first place. During medical school itself, if they are keen, they often do further research, or may actually pursue MD-PhD programmes in which research is an integral part. Some medical schools in the USA and now in Australia also offer a period of dedicated time to pursue research usually lasting around one year. During this year, they can undertake a small project which leads to a small thesis and often one or two publications. Again, this research helps set them up to get into a good speciality training programme. In the USA and to a lesser extent in Australia, trainees in speciality training programmes often complete small projects that lead to research publications during that time, again with the understanding that further research and publications is likely to get them a better fellowship position. The latter entail one or two years of subspeciality training within the basic speciality training programme; for example, a year of hand surgery training after a basic orthopaedic surgery training. Candidates for these sub-speciality training programmes are more attractive if they have published a number of papers. In turn, in the USA, Australia and the UK, research during such sub-speciality fellowship training is common and is often a very productive time.

In the USA the major research degree is a PhD, which is indeed highly valued. It is usually completed after a basic science degree before medical school or during medical school as part of an MD-PhD programme. Nevertheless, in the USA, a specific research degree carries less value than it does in the UK and Australia. Instead, potential employers look more closely at the actual publication record.

Summary
- Deciding when to do research is an important, but difficult, decision.
- There are a number of options, each with their own advantages and disadvantages.
- When you choose to do research will depend on both your personal and professional circumstances.

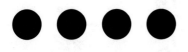

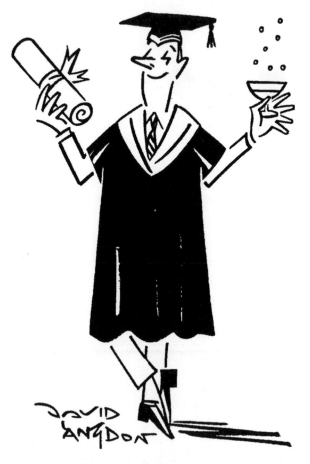

Higher degree . . .

4

Selecting a research degree

Most medics doing a period of research will wish to work for a higher university degree. Besides the intrinsic interest they will have in pursuing such research, they will be balancing the time they will be putting aside for this against the benefits such an exercise would confer for their future careers.

What degrees are available?

Some UK and Commonwealth universities encourage their medical (undergraduate) students to enter for intercalated Bachelor of Medical Science (BMedSc) or Bachelor of Science (BSc) degrees. Others offer postgraduate Master of Philosophy (MPhil) or Master of Science (MSc) degrees. At the postgraduate level, most universities offer a Doctorate of Philosophy (PhD or DPhil). Some US and UK universities have combined MD-PhD and MB-PhD programmes. Most universities in the UK and Commonwealth also offer MD (Doctor or Medicine) and MS (Master of Surgery) degrees for medical and surgical candidates, respectively. In London, the MD and MS have now been replaced by the MD(Res) (Doctor of Medicine (Research)) degree. Other universities have abandoned the MS and, at these universities, the surgical candidates submit an MD thesis alongside their medical colleagues, and are subject to the same regulations. The standard (and often the regulations) for the degree of MS and MD are considered to be equivalent to each other. Note that in the US, the MD (Doctorate of Medicine) is the basic medical degree, not a higher research-based medical degree.

The intercalated BSc

In the UK, Oxford and Cambridge students have compulsory third-year courses, usually including a research module, which lead to an Honours BA. At most other universities, an extra year's course (which is usually taken as a third year), is optional and leads to an Honours BSc or BMedSc. It is important for the student to consult university regulations, discuss the advantages and disadvantages of pursuing such a course with senior students and take the advice of the course supervisor before taking the important decision of whether or not to apply for this course. Do not do it just to get some letters after your name! You should have a definite interest in the particular subject (anatomy, pathology or whatever), and a genuine desire both to study the subject at greater depth and to carry out a research project. If not, you may find your third year is frustrating and dull, especially when you see your colleagues enjoying life as clinical students with their newly acquired stethoscopes around their necks.

Courses vary from university to university and from subject to subject. Normally, they comprise a number of modules, one of which involves research. For example, the BSc in Clinical Anatomy at King's College, London, with which one of us (Harold Ellis) is involved, is made up of a course of lectures and demonstrations in clinical anatomy, a dissection with presentation to the outside examiner, and a research project. Few students at this stage will have a particular research project in mind and thus rely on choosing the topics from a list provided by the course supervisor.

Doctor of Medicine (MD or DM)

Clinical candidates typically opt for the Doctor of Medicine. To be eligible, candidates are generally required to have held a primary medical degree of the university concerned for a minimum of two to five years and to be fully registered or hold limited registration with the General Medical Council. The stringency of additional requirements varies with university. Some universities used to require candidates to hold their own primary medical degree, but most now accept applicants who hold any registrable primary qualification. Oxford and Cambridge Universities, however, still require candidates to hold one of their primary degrees (this includes the BA), as well as a registrable medical qualification. An MD thesis usually deals with a topic in medicine, or any branch of medicine, or medical science. It typically embodies original findings, and observes certain conditions of presentation and overall length. In addition, candidates are frequently examined *viva voce*.

Most universities advise their candidates to seek more senior advice in the field covered by the proposed thesis at an early stage. Some universities exceptionally allow a submission in the form of previously published work rather than a thesis.

Master of Surgery (MS)

The Master of Surgery is more popular with surgical candidates, although some now opt for the MD. Again, typically, the candidate must have held a medical degree for not less than five years, and have spent not less than two years in training posts in surgery or in a special branch of surgery approved by one of the Royal Colleges of Surgery, and be fully registered with the General Medical Council. As with the MD, Oxford and Cambridge Universities additionally require candidates to hold one of their primary degrees. The thesis would deal with a topic in general surgery or with some special branch of surgery, and there may also be an oral examination.

Doctor of Philosophy (PhD or DPhil)

Regulations for PhD degrees are even more varied between universities. These usually entail residence and full-time research in the university over stipulated times (two to four years; not less than three years in the University of Cambridge). This degree cannot normally be attempted while simultaneously holding a primarily clinical attachment, but many doctors choose to continue a limited amount of on-call or clinic work. Some universities offer part-time PhD programmes. However, registration for a PhD usually only requires a first degree and does not require full clinical qualifications as demanded by MD or MS regulations. Thus, one can begin work for a PhD immediately after one's primary medical qualification or intercalated BSc. Some universities are also now offering four year PhD programmes where the first year entails three four-month placements in different laboratories to acquire different research skills before choosing one of the areas of research to continue in for the following three years.

PhD theses are extremely varied and range from pure laboratory research or even mathematical modelling away from the laboratory bench to clinical trials. The format you choose will depend on both your level of training and your particular area of interest.

Shorter degree courses (MSc, MPhil, etc.) usually also stipulate a period of full-time work resident in the university and can be taken very soon after one's primary qualification.

Choosing a degree

The degree one attempts depends on a number of factors. These include:

- the time required for completion,
- your own qualifications,
- individual university regulations,
- prestige,

- funding available,
- the subject matter you wish to study, and
- the country in which you wish to work.

Time required for completion

You will certainly have views about the length of time you wish to devote to research, and this will influence what you attempt. A doctorate is the most substantial qualification, but takes a longer time. Examples of completion times for postgraduate degrees include:

Bachelor of Medical Science (BMedSc)	1 year
Intercalated Bachelor of Science (BSc)	1 year
Master of Philosophy (MPhil)	1–2 years
Master of Science (MSc)	1–2 years
Doctor of Medicine (MD or DM)	2–3 years
Master of Surgery (MS or MCh)	2–3 years
Doctor of Medicine (Research) (MD(Res))	2–3 years
Doctor of Philosophy (PhD or DPhil)	3–4 years

Your own qualifications

Your entry to a higher degree requires acceptance by both the university and the department in which you wish to work. The level of degree for which your application would be eligible will vary with your own academic background and track record within it. In the UK, studentships, scholarships and fellowships for which you may apply for financial support often require an honours degree with a II.1 or higher final grade, and both an MD and MS require you to have completed a primary medical degree. In addition, you need to check particular regulations very carefully: many universities only allow their own graduates to attempt their higher degrees, particularly medical doctorates. Other universities allow external applications.

Individual university regulations

Different universities vary widely in their regulations and requirements, even for equivalent higher degrees. It is therefore important to check such details with the admissions office or the postgraduate dean of your prospective university, particularly if it is not your undergraduate university. You should also study carefully the postgraduate prospectuses, to get an idea of available departments, and the research areas they offer. The scope and quality of postgraduate research varies greatly between universities, and even between departments in the same university. Finally, it is prudent to seek advice from someone who has recently embarked on the programme you are considering, once you become interested in a particular department.

Prestige

A PhD is considered by some to carry the most scientific weight. Some medical circles may regard an MD or MS as more relevant, especially for a future career in a branch of clinical medicine or surgery.

Funding available

Most universities charge fees when one is working in residence for a higher academic degree. If you have a grant or scholarship to cover such expenses, consider attempting the longer, more prestigious degree. If you are self-funded, a shorter, less expensive higher medical degree may be more practical.

The subject matter you wish to study

There are usually relatively few restrictions concerning exact subject matter for higher degrees, but each university has its own particular regulations. A PhD, MSc or BMedSc is often orientated more towards basic sciences, while an MD or MS is more clinically biased in subject matter. However, overlap can and does occur and so many MD or MS theses are entirely laboratory-based, although one would expect these latter to have some clinical relevance.

The country where you wish to work

In the USA and Canada the major research degree is a PhD. It is usually a four-year degree that involves a considerable amount of course work in the early stages. Australia has similar options to those in the UK: in other words, an undergraduate research degree, a MD/MS or a PhD.

Summary

- There are a number of available research degrees within medicine.
- Which degree is right for you depends on a number of factors, including how long you want to spend on research, your own qualifications and the available funding.

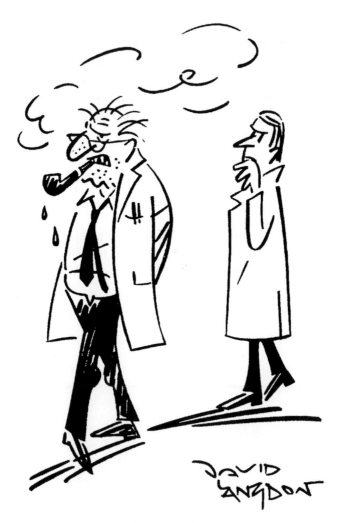

Your supervisor . . .

5

Choosing a department, research supervisor and project

After deciding on the timing for your research programme and the degree to which you wish to aspire, you next need to decide where you would like to conduct your research, whom you would like to work with and what you are going to work on. The order in which you decide these and their relative importance will vary significantly between individuals and specific circumstances. It might be that before you actually start applying for research positions, you have strong ideas about the area of research you might pursue, and the person with whom you may wish to work. If that is the case, it will determine the channels along which you will make enquiries and applications. Alternatively you may seek openings or scholarships at particular departments with initially less specific interests in mind, and seek a direction for your research afterwards. Most applicants will discover a middle course, being initially drawn towards a broad area of research and a department, then gradually acquiring knowledge of available research projects and personnel as enquiries and the application proceed. In this latter case, a good place to start is a university or clinical department whose work or interest lies close to interests in your desired career path. For instance, if you would like ultimately to be a transplant surgeon, you might try the local university department of surgery. If your career plans have not yet crystallized, the decision is inevitably more difficult.

Whichever process you take, there are a few common areas to consider during this important process.

Exploring departments and universities

It is prudent to learn a little about any particular department, or University, you are considering. You should think about trying the following.

1. A computer search to find the range and scope of publications produced over recent years by that department.
2. Talking to previous students who have worked in that department. This is invaluable. It could provide you with detailed information about the areas being studied, and about the scientists who work there.
3. Consulting a more senior colleague, who is now in the kind of position you would like eventually to achieve yourself, about the academic and research standing of that department. It can come as a surprise later in your career to find out how important the research standing of your chosen department is.

The function of your research supervisor

Your supervisor is the senior member in the research group to whom you will be assigned, and who will provide guidance in the course of your research project. He or she will be the most important individual to your academic well-being during your time in research. He or she is likely to be someone who has research experience and who can provide the assistance and advice you need to make progress. In general, these should include:

- the equipment and materials you will need;
- initial ideas;
- general research knowledge;
- knowledge specific to the topic you will be investigating;
- technical expertise;

- a critical reader as your written work starts to appear, who will make thoughtful and constructive comments, not only about the work you have done, but also the quality of your writing;
- a 'clock': your supervisor should give you indications of your progress, and encourage you to present your work to specific meetings at the appropriate time;
- an introduction to other researchers with knowledge beyond his or her own should this prove necessary; and
- an introduction to future employers.

The process is not all one way. In return, your supervisor is likely to receive:

- inexpensive research labour;
- your own knowledge, both original and acquired;
- your ideas, ingenuity, energy and time; and
- an expansion of his or her net research activity, with publications in collaboration with you.

There are three ways to obtain a supervisor.

1. The prospective supervisor approaches you.
2. You approach the supervisor.
3. The head of the department assigns you to a particular supervisor.

Choosing your research supervisor

The choice of supervisor is, perhaps, the most important and most difficult of your decisions. There is a good deal of luck involved in terms of the fit of personalities and ideas. If you do not like the look of your potential supervisor, it is best to decide upon a change of supervisor at an early stage, rather than offending him or her and many others later. Perhaps to be initially non-committal is an advantage. On the one hand, it goes without saying that you need a supervisor with the expertise in the subject in which you are interested, in order to complete your research successfully. On the other, the fit between individuals within the supervisor–student relationship will have a profound effect on the success of your research activities. Within limits, therefore, it is probably more desirable to compromise an apparently more desirable project for a supervisor whom you feel confident can lead your research development, even if in a slightly different subject area.

The relationship between a supervisor and their research student is a subtle one, and dealing with later breakdowns in this relationship, should these occur, are difficult and distressing for all concerned. Such a state of affairs can result from situations when the research project appears to be going badly, there are divergent scientific interests of opinion, clashes of personality and approach, or mixtures of these.

It is difficult to predict precisely how supervision turns out, but at the very least, to cover these major eventualities, you will need to make an assessment about (1) the research interests and research capacity of your prospective supervisor, (2) the extent to which you feel you can work together, and (3) the laboratory, department and university that provides the backdrop for this relationship.

1. If you have a say in the matter, the departmental head or secretary can provide a list of academics within the department. It will be useful to check on their publications and to talk to their previous research students. This will give you an idea of a particular supervisor's fields of interest, the size of his or her research group, the degree of contact he or she offers within the laboratory, and the extent to which their research is successful as evidenced in their publication output. This advice may appear peculiar, but if you do not feel convinced about the scientific ability and competence of your supervisor, it is unlikely that your project will proceed smoothly!

2. Individuals vary greatly in their approach to supervision. At one extreme, you may find groups in which individuals work closely with their supervisor. This is particularly the case in

small research groups. This offers the benefits of their direct input into your work, and a closer interest in whether experimental and analysis techniques are being effectively learnt and correctly performed. However, your supervisor may then have a more direct input into the ideas that you choose to pursue, and a closer micromanagement of your research direction. At the other extreme, supervisors may have relatively little contact with their research students, leaving much of the day-to-day development of their projects in the hands of postdoctoral research workers, particularly in large research groups. This may leave you more free to pursue some of your detailed interests, but you may then feel isolated in your work, and feel that this remoteness defeats the purpose of working with a particular individual! The majority of supervisors are likely to pursue an intermediate course, taking greater interest in your initial development, and then leaving you with some freedom to chart your own detailed research direction.

3. The backdrop behind the supervisor–student relationship is formed by particular features of his or her laboratory, and the department and university in which you work. These also vary greatly in the extent and nature of the institutional support they offer their students. This should include arrangements for some form of mentorship in which an additional faculty member can provide advice and encouragement and support. More minor but useful means of assistance include support for travel costs to conferences at the departmental level. Most universities now run postgraduate courses covering scientific fundamentals such as statistical methods, safety practices in laboratories, and basic scientific practice such as the maintenance of experimental records at the departmental or faculty level.

It is thus difficult to evaluate all the pros and cons of particular supervisors in particular laboratories or departments in a limited set of meetings, but at the very least, it is wise to contact or write to prospective supervisors to arrange meetings and to see their laboratory. This meeting will form a useful means of mutual assessment.

Choosing a research topic

The overall topic which you choose to research will depend on a number of factors

1. Your own interests and aspirations.
2. Whether you prefer team vs. individual work.
3. Your supervisor's interests.
4. Facilities available in the department.
5. Whether you wish to work on experimental or human systems.

1. Considering your own interests and aspirations

Clearly, if you wish to become a neurosurgeon, you will be more interested in examining 'the effects of nerve growth factor in the sensory cortex' than the 'morphogenesis of bone cells'. However, it is not always possible to get very close to your true interest. This is usually due to limitations of physical, technical or academic expertise. In these cases, you need to weigh up the advantages of expertise with its greater guarantee of success and the potentially more exciting but dangerous individualism.

2. Team vs. individual work

An important but often forgotten consideration in choosing your research area is the amount of independence you want. There are a wide range of research laboratories. Large teams often have nearly everyone working on the same project. This has the advantage that your research is likely to be completed, but you may feel a very small cog in a big machine, and your name may only be one of many to appear on the research papers. Molecular biological research tends to be expensive and to involve large, salaried teams. At the other extreme, working in some areas of cellular electrophysiology involves groups of as few as one or two scientists, and entails a lonelier existence. However, the research tends to be inexpensive, and the resulting published work involves few authors.

3. Your supervisor's interests

It is likely that you will have something in mind regarding your research project. Your supervisor will also have a project in mind. The two may not always coincide. It is likely that both you and your supervisor will be constrained by research commitments that arise out of his funding. In general, it is advisable initially to follow your supervisor's ideas as he is more likely to have the research knowledge to make more informed, realistic decisions. As your work and reading progress, you will acquire the knowledge and skills to become more independent. Most supervisors will encourage this independence at the appropriate time.

In this way, the relationship between research supervisor and student is very much like a parent–child one. Most initial decisions and overall care, including funding and housing, are provided by the parent. As the child matures, he is able to make more of his own decisions and please his parents with signs of independence. Nevertheless, the parental figure should always be there to 'rescue' the child in times of unforeseen hardship. Conversely, the child will be more productive and less obstreperous if given the freedom (at the correct time) to pursue his own interests. The relationship may then become synergistic, in which both parties learn and gain from the relationship. The parent–child analogy follows through many aspects of the supervisor–supervisee relationship, including an occasional lack of objectivity on the part of both the student and the supervisor!

4. Considering the facilities available

However good your reason for wishing to pursue a particular area, this will be frustrated if your research group does not have the requisite facilities, background or personnel. Your research area will consequently be affected by a number of practical limitations. These include the following:

1. *Laboratory workshop facilities.* A limited number of these (whether providing mechanical, electrical engineering or tissue culture support), will be available and well established in your laboratory. It is prudent to work on a project *whereby* demands will be realistic in relation to what your supporting department technicians are accustomed to, as you will then have a source of help when in difficulty.

2. *Expertise available.* Quite clearly, it would be most prudent to work on areas where your supervisor and his colleagues have experience and expertise. At all events, major departures from this norm must not be undertaken lightly and are risky for the inexperienced scientist.

3. *Time available.* It is unrealistic to expect to develop a substantial new technique in a limited time. In contrast, someone holding a longer-term position may try projects in areas in which the research group may not have experience.

4. *Cost and funding.* In general, it is more practical and efficient to confine your experiments to those for which your laboratory is already equipped. Frequently, your supervisor will have taken you on a grant with fairly specific provisions and terms of reference that may not readily allow for major departures in direction.

5. *Your own expertise.* Under certain circumstances, you may have already acquired expertise in a particular technique elsewhere. You might then consider trying such a technique even if this is novel to your present research group. However, you must bear in mind that setting up new procedures may be unexpectedly time-consuming in a different environment,

and this extra time must justify itself in terms of interest or results.

6. *Subjects.* You will need something or someone upon which to conduct your research. In general terms, medical research can be conducted on (1) cells and tissues, (2) animals, or (3) humans. Different departments or laboratories will have different capacities in these areas. Each system has its own advantages and disadvantages; some of these are briefly commented on below.

Human medical research

Research involving humans is often thought to be the most obviously applicable to clinical medicine. There are several approaches to studying human populations. These include the following:

1. *Observation or intervention.* You may simply observe particular phenomena in your human subjects; for example, the proportion of patients with a palmaris longus tendon in a population of patients with and without Dupuytren's contracture. Alternatively, you may conduct a clinical trial, where one form of intervention or management is assessed against another; for example, the effect of total mastectomy with or without radiotherapy on the five-year survival of patients with breast cancer.

2. *Population studies.* A study may describe a single case of a given condition or treatment (e.g. the first splenic transplant), a sample of a given population, or the whole population (e.g. the incidence of skin cancer in Faeroe Islanders).

3. *Prospective or retrospective trials.* A prospective study makes an initial assessment on a given population and then follows up the same group over a period of time. A retrospective study looks backwards in time, after the event; for example, looking up the case notes of patients with lung cancer diagnosed by bronchoscopy.

4. *Controlled versus uncontrolled trials.* A simple control group is one which omits the 'active treatment', but is otherwise identical in every way to the treatment group. Control groups can be more sophisticated and include patients treated with the 'standard' drug or combinations of new and old treatments. For a controlled trial to be valid, patients need to be allocated to the control and treatment groups in a randomized fashion.

5. Research involving patients must allow for the appreciable time required to complete protocols. For example, a prospective trial requires patients to be collected, the procedure studied to be completed, and then a suitable period allowed to elapse for review. Will this be a practical proposition for the amount of time you have available? If not, think again! You may have to restrict your plans to investigating a population that has already been documented and is awaiting continuing detailed analysis and study rather than starting entirely from scratch. Indeed, this latter option is probably the most frequent clinical research project to be allocated to you if your available research time is fairly limited.

6. *Cadaveric human material.* The dissecting room of the department of anatomy and the autopsy room of the department of pathology provide a wealth of material which is available for research. This has the great advantage of almost immediate availability. Of course, this will require permission of the department head and the collaboration of the technical staff. Examples of recent studies in the dissecting room carried out by research students and demonstrators under the supervision of one of us (Harold Ellis) include: the gross and histological study of the thymus gland in the elderly; the incidence of aortic aneurysm at post-mortem; variations in the tortuosity of the splenic artery and its relationship to age; the distribution of valves in the gonadal veins; and the 'zone of danger' of the accessory nerve in operations on the posterior triangle of the neck.

7. *Pathological tissues.* The pathology department, especially at a university hospital, will almost certainly have a rich collection of preserved pathological tissues, and further materials will be continually forthcoming from the operating theatres and the autopsy room. With modern staining techniques, especially those applied for example to immunofluorescence, this superb source of research is not to be neglected.

8. *Radiological and imaging material.* The radiological department is another excellent area for research. Again, you will need the permission of the department director, the help and advice of a sympathetic radiologist who has a particular interest in your subject, and the co-operation of the secretarial staff. All this having been obtained, valuable studies can be instituted with all the advantages of the immediately available material. Again, examples from our own recent experience include studies on variations in the size of the colon in different ethnic groups using double-contrast barium enema X-rays, variations in the anatomy of the superior mediastinum using computerized tomography, and variations of the spinal cord and dural theca levels using magnetic resonance imaging (MRI).

Experimental systems

Research using animal models is usually simpler and quicker, but may appear less immediately clinically applicable. However, the scientist then has greater control over the experiment and subjects. In any case, new drugs or operative procedures must be tested on animal models before human trials. For such experiments, animal house facilities within, or available to, the department are essential. If you are considering working with animals, it is worth noting the following:

1. Animal houses are very expensive to set up. They must fulfil strict criteria for the humane management of animals

controlled by law, and regulated as designated establishments (in the UK) by the Home Office.

2. Animals must be obtained from reputable suppliers, recognized as such by the Home Office.

3. Research Grants will normally allow you the recurrent costs of purchasing and maintaining the animal, but no more.

4. Overhead costs of animal house facilities, apart from board and lodging, usually cannot be met from a grant.

The study of cultured or otherwise isolated cells and tissues in vitro offers even greater powers of manipulation to the researchers. However, the results obtained are not necessarily applicable in vivo (in the living organism). In addition, the time necessary to prepare or grow the cells to conduct meaningful experiments varies with species of animal and with cell type. Tissue culture and other in vitro cellular work requires its own services and infrastructure within the department.

Ethical aspects

Your own ethical views and belief systems must be reconciled to the nature of the work you are planning to pursue, and must be clear to the individuals with whom you seek to work before taking on a research position.

The ethics of working on human subjects is a large and important area of discussion. Most clinical trials must have prior approval from the local (usually hospital) ethical committee. It is important to determine at an early stage whether such approval is necessary and to initiate the procedures entailed, as the process can take many months. Most countries also have set criteria for carrying out drug trials. In the UK, a doctor or dentist is considered to be carrying out a clinical trial if he administers a medicinal product primarily to determine its effect. The doctor is then required to have a clinical trials certificate, or the manufacturer to hold a product licence.

A number of important regulations apply to animal experimentation to ensure that the most humane procedures possible are used in scientific work. The precise details by which these controls are applied vary with state or with country. They need to be studied carefully before contemplating animal research. Such controls are applied according to conditions and guidelines set by national scrutinizing bodies; for example, the Home Office in the UK or the National Research Council in the US.

In the UK, permission to perform animal experiments is covered by the Animals (Scientific Procedures) Act 1986 (which covers all vertebrates, *Octopus vulgaris*, and foetal and larval forms beyond certain stages of development), under which licences are issued. Every individual researcher who wishes to conduct procedures that fall outside a restricted range of manipulations must apply for a *Personal Licence*. This can be applied for once you have taken approved courses and passed a qualifying examination in the procedures on the animal species on which you wish to work. A *Project Licence* is also required. This is issued to institutions that are recognized as designated establishments which conduct scientific work. Applications for these require the project to be described, and the procedures on any living animal involved to be defined. Your institution may already have project licences to cover your intended project and its contained procedures for which further application is then not necessary. Information on Home Office Licences is obtainable from the Home Office Inspector responsible for the institution in which you propose to carry out your research.

In vitro studies of human tissues, including clinical material, require permission of the consultant in charge and written informed consent from the patients concerned. Sacrifice of animals in order to obtain tissues for in vitro study should conform to the Code of Practice for the Humane Killing of Animals under Schedule 1 to the Animals (Scientific Procedures) Act 1986, in the UK, or equivalent legislation in other countries. Where a method is used that is not included in Schedule 1, this must be permitted under a pre-existing Home Office licence.

The researcher who proposes to use patients for research owes a particular moral duty towards them. This is elaborated in codified terms in the World Medical Association Declaration of Helsinki (last modified 1996) and, in the UK, in the Medical Research Council document on Responsibility in Investigations on Human Participants and Material and on Personal Information (1992). Patients who volunteer for such research can face risks over and above those normally encountered in their everyday lives. A volunteer competent to do so should choose whether or not to participate after being given correct information about the nature, purpose and duration of the experiment; the methods and means by which it is conducted; all inconveniences and hazards reasonably to be expected; and the effects upon health or person which may possibly come from his or her participation in the experiment. It is hardly necessary to say that volunteers should not be subjected to any force or coercion and that they are free to withdraw at any time without jeopardy.

To deny volunteers such information is a clear breach of their moral rights. However, this moral emphasis on informed consent is backed up by the law. Legally, a battery is committed if volunteers who participate in medical research are touched without being provided with adequate information about what the researcher proposes to do and why. Specific circumstances under which different interventions under investigation will be offered should also be communicated, for example, whether the participants will be randomized in the study. A researcher will be deemed negligent if he or she does not adhere to the professional duty to communicate adequate information about risks and here the standard of disclosure is even higher than for ordinary routine treatment. A prudent research worker should warn volunteers of risks in the detail that any 'reasonable person' would require. Informed consent in research with children must always be obtained from someone with parental authority.

If you are proposing to use patients for your research, we strongly advise you to read a most useful article by Professor Len

Doyle entitled 'Informed consent in medical research' (*British Medical Journal* 1997, **314**, pp. 1107–11), which also gives a list of interesting references for further reading.

Summary
- How you choose a department, research supervisor and project will depend on your individual circumstances, but a common path is to be initially drawn to a broad area of research and a department and then, in time, to a specific supervisor and project.
- Choosing a supervisor is, perhaps, the most important and most difficult of your decisions.
- Consider arranging meetings with prospective supervisors and speaking to others who have been supervised by them before.
- Think carefully about your topic of research, the methods you wish to use and the systems, whether human or experimental, upon which you intend to work.

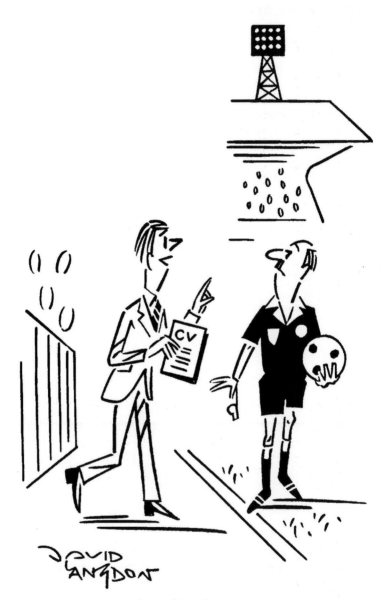

Approaching referees ...

6

Applying for research positions and funding

Having decided on a particular department or research unit, and having confirmed that it offers research opportunities, either through a postgraduate programme or advertisements of research positions, you may consider making an application. This entails:

- obtaining further background information about the department or position,
- setting out information about yourself in the form of a curriculum vitae,
- finding referees who will write about you, and
- applying for funding.

Background information about the available position

Before applying for any position you need to find out about the selection procedure. This information will usually be available from the departmental secretary, postgraduate tutor or departmental website. In particular, it is worth finding out:

- who is on the selection committee;
- the closing date for applications;
- how many candidates will be short listed;
- the date, place, time and length of interview;
- how many candidates will be selected and how many posts are available; and
- when the decision will be announced.

Visiting your future place of employment is also important, particularly when deciding upon a research supervisor or if you are already interested in one. Many departments will prefer candidates who have already approached, and been regarded as acceptable for, research supervision by a particular staff member. Talk with those who have been or who are already there, ask about the work conducted there, possible supervisors, etc.

Your curriculum vitae

You next need to furnish information about yourself to your possible future employers. Although most medical jobs now require applicants to complete a standard application form, most candidates for research positions are still asked to submit a curriculum vitae. Your curriculum vitae is thus the major means by which you convey details about yourself in postgraduate research applications and, in some cases, may be the only thing your potential employers see before drawing up a short list for the interview. It is accordingly imperative to give the best account of yourself.

The following particulars must be included in a curriculum vitae.

1. Name.
2. Address, telephone number, e-mail.
3. Date of birth.
4. Nationality.
5. Current and previous positions held.
6. School education.
7. University education.
8. Qualifications (with class, or honours, if relevant) with dates.
9. Scholarships, prizes and academic awards.
10. Positions of responsibility in chronological order.
11. Membership of professional organizations.
12. Publications.

13. Interests and hobbies.
14. Names and addresses of referees.

It is also worth enclosing a covering letter. This should ideally be only one page and include a paragraph summarizing your educational background, achievements and future objectives.

Approaching referees

Most job applications require you to supply names (and addresses) of two or three referees. They should preferably be:

- previous employers or teachers who know you and your work well;
- in fields relevant to your application;
- people whom you believe to have a good opinion of your own work and academic performance.

Once you have decided which referees you want:

1. Write to them asking if they would support your application.
2. Send them a copy of your application, including curriculum vitae and a summary of what you have done since they were last in contact with you.
3. Give them a brief account of the position for which you are applying.
4. Let them know the eventual outcome of your application, thanking them, particularly if you are successful.

Your funding requirements

You need to think about the following financial implications of pursuing a period of research. These divide into salary requirements, fee costs and the cost of the research itself.

1. You will need a stipend to cover your own *salary needs* during your period of research. From your own personal point of view, it is important to bear in mind that in general, research

positions offer considerably lower stipends than do full-time clinical appointments and so periods in full-time research entail significant financial sacrifice.

2. A considerable *fee component* may be payable in the case of MSc, MPhil and PhD degrees. However, the time when one can attempt a PhD or MSc in relation to one's qualification date is flexible. In the UK and Commonwealth, the MD and MS are usually taken as career degrees and so recurrent fees are usually not charged. In addition, apart from a require-ment for full medical qualification, the regulations regarding completion time, subject and supervisor for these latter two higher degrees are less tight. If, at the outset, you decide upon a one-year MSc course, bear in mind that it may not be possi-ble to 'upgrade' this to a PhD should you wish to do so in the course of the work, and the year in which you are supported may still be deducted from subsequent research support by some funding councils.

3. If you are conducting research as a postgraduate student or as a candidate for a higher medical degree, *research expenses* are usually covered by your supervisor's grant or by the labora-tory. Accordingly, you will normally have to think relatively little about research costs other than your own applications for fellowships and studentships for your own personal support.

Applying for funding

Research and postgraduate work is funded by a range of pri-vate charities and government agencies that vary within each country. It is highly likely you will be applying competitively to one of these either directly or indirectly through the department to which you will be making applications. The following observa-tions may be helpful:

1. You should familiarize yourself with the agencies available to offer support. In the UK, there is a wide range of specialist

charitable organizations in addition to relatively large organizations that fund research on a national scale. Of these, government agencies include the Medical Research Council (MRC), the Biotechnology and Biological Sciences Research Council (BBSRC), the Engineering and Physical Sciences Research Council (EPSRC) and the National Environmental Research Council (NERC). Important private charities with a large input into research at the national level include the Wellcome Trust and British Heart Foundation (BHF). Each has its own terms of reference, and particular interests. All have websites that provide indications of the support they have to offer, and vary in the generosity and adequacy of their support.

2. You should thoroughly familiarize yourself with what each agency offers, and take careful notes of their closing dates and time elapsed between receipt of application and final decision.

3. You should be aware that applications are highly competitive, and application to more than one agency, depending on closing and decision dates, would be highly prudent.

4. Applications for positions are also often complex, and require a co-ordination between yourself and your possible supervisor, with both needing to fill in details at particular times.

5. Both closing and decision dates often occur at fixed times during the year, and you will want to have produced and submitted an application in good time if you wish to time the start of your research strategically in relationship to the sequence of your clinical attachments.

6. The precise nature of your possible funding by any of these organizations varies considerably with the stage at which you wish to enter research. In general, those entering research immediately following the undergraduate or qualification level can apply for grants and scholarships. In many cases, quotas of these are awarded to particular universities and departments to be made available for competition. These

include studentships for both three or four years (frequently PhD), one or two years (frequently MPhil or MSc degrees), as well as the PhD components of MB-PhD programmes. These often cover costs of the fee component of the postgraduate course, together with a stipend. In either case your supervisor will require his own grant funding to cover the actual costs of your research.

7. Those who have proceeded further in clinical medicine, particularly following their first postgraduate clinical examinations, and especially those who have been successfully selected for further specialist training (ST3 onwards) can be eligible for highly competitive Medical Research Council or Wellcome Trust clinical training fellowships. These entail providing detailed research proposals that you will need to discuss with your prospective supervisor. Such awards often cover costs of the fee component for the postgraduate course, together with a stipend, and contributions to the actual costs of the research itself. Extensive preparation is needed in applying for these awards, and so it will be prudent to explore these well before any closing dates.

8. It is possible that a supervisor may have grant funding for his research that may provide salary support for you to act as a research assistant, but often the fee component of your course will have to come from this salary.

Applying for research positions overseas

Graduate programmes in the USA are considerably more organized than in the UK, with explicitly advertised courses and periods of research. It is often therefore necessary to apply in a more formal way, usually on forms with instructions obtained from the dean of the graduate school. Applications usually have to be accompanied by an 'academic transcript' and confidential letters of evaluation, sent directly to the graduate school. Depending on the admitting departments, American candidates often additionally take Graduate Record Examination (GRE) general and subject tests. It is likely that a foreign candidate, particularly a British honours degree holder, may have such requirements modified. However, other foreign students, particularly those from non-English speaking countries, may have to satisfy further language requirements. This typically involves a certification of English proficiency from the Test of English as a Foreign Language (TOEFL). You may also have to produce statements confirming your financial ability to support a course of graduate study.

Owing to the more formal nature of American graduate courses, it is essential that all information is sent to the university graduate school office well before the specified deadlines. Preliminary enquiries, particularly in heavily subscribed universities, may have to begin several years before the projected starting date.

American students sometimes pursue graduate work on a part-time basis. However, this is not permitted for overseas students by visa regulations.

Overseas graduate students face a number of additional expenses in the US, with which the UK graduate, for example, may not be familiar. A full-time graduate student pays a university fee every semester, although this is reduced for individuals simultaneously working as teaching or research assistants. Cover must also be arranged for accident and sickness insurance. Your financial support must also cover registration, student health fees and apartment rents, in addition to meals, books and other personal expenses.

Some financial assistance is available even within US universities as fellowships and scholarships, but US Federal programmes tend to support US citizens and permanent residents only. Individual departments may offer paid graduate and research assistantships. US research degrees entail substantial course work, and satisfactory performance at associated examinations, and therefore differ substantially from British graduate curricula.

Information on times and places of graduate record examinations may be obtained from:

Education Testing Service, PO Box 6000, Princeton, NJ 08541–6000, USA

Information on Test of English as a Foreign Language (TOEFL) may be obtained from:

Educational Testing Service, PO Box 6155, Princeton, NJ 08541–6155, USA

Summary

- Applying for a research position involves a number of vital steps.
- Before applying for a research position, visit potential departments and talk to others working or who have worked there.
- Establish the funding situation.

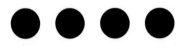

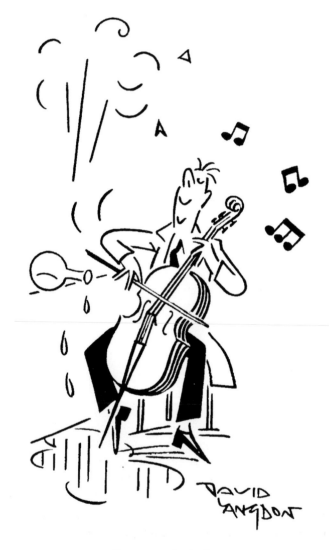

Extracurricular buffer…

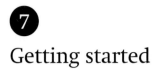

Getting started

The first phase: getting started

Congratulations! You have now passed the major initial hurdles of making the decision to pursue research, and of following this decision through to the position where you are able to start. The remarks in this chapter primarily concern your fitting into, and learning to function in, this new environment. How you begin your period of research and the methods you use will obviously vary depending on whether your research is primarily laboratory or patient based. There are, however, many issues common to all types of research.

A doctor in research

When you join a research group, whether in a university or clinical department, you will find yourself in a very different setting, with values distinct from those to which you are accustomed in the clinic or ward. You should try as quickly as possible to assimilate into the local scene. Even if the atmosphere is initially alien to you, this may reflect its tradition of research achievement just as the particular environment in a successful hospital promotes good clinical results. However, this does not mean a clinician does not have anything to offer a research environment. Some of the advantages you will have gained from a clinical background are as follows:

- You will often be more realistic as to what to expect of others.
- You will often have more social confidence and take more care in your dealings with others.

- You will have a better sense of what can or cannot be achieved in limited time.
- You will have gained more experience in making full use of available time.
- You are more used to coping with more than one problem at a time.
- You can often assist scientific colleagues with your ability to gain access to clinical material or knowledge.

However, there are a number of respects in which you must adapt:

- You may be used to responding only to well-defined authority figures. In a research environment such individuals are not as clear-cut.
- You may feel less confident at the bench. When starting out you will often find yourself embarrassingly out of touch with even elementary scientific procedures.
- You may expect too much of the services of others.
- You may be less accustomed to the longer-term planning that goes with research work.

Public relations

It follows that, as a fledgling researcher, you will depend greatly on the goodwill and the skills of others, and upon your relationships with key people. As in medicine, it is therefore important to establish and maintain a good rapport with everyone in the department, whether scientific, technical, secretarial or administrative staff. You should aim to establish yourself as someone who is seen to be:

- diligent and productive;
- honest;
- courteous (for example, keep appointments and, if away, leave a note with a contact number or time of return on your desk);
- reliable with colleagues and with the use of delicate apparatus and potentially costly reagents;
- likely to benefit from any assistance given;
- grateful for assistance (for example, consider giving small Christmas presents, or at least cards, to your laboratory technician,

secretary, and anyone else who has given you significant assistance over the year); and

- likely to acknowledge assistance received (for example, you might send copies of your publications with acknowledgements to those who gave you help).

An example of how good relations will smooth your time in research is your association with the technical department. By placing small, simple, non-urgent requests with the department early, it is unlikely that you will need to harass the staff and you will be genuinely grateful when the equipment returns or is repaired well in advance of your deadline. Furthermore, by establishing good rapport, the technical staff would then be more receptive when you have genuinely urgent or difficult demands, for example, in relation to completing a paper or performing experiments in response to a referee's report.

Self-discipline

Research requires ample amounts of both self-assurance and self-control. You must be strict with yourself and be realistic with use of your time in relation to your ultimate aims. Research work is usually very individualistic; the success or failure of your project depends primarily upon yourself. Conversely, a lot of the other people in your department are tied to more formal commitments, so you should also feel free to study in the library, write at home, or take a short sporting or holiday break if you know it will help you achieve your goal. Nevertheless, in the absence of other factors, it is best to keep regular and consistent hours of work, at times when help and colleagues are available.

Maintaining clinical commitments

There is great value in maintaining a 'clinical string to your bow', particularly during longer stints in research (greater than six months). Consider the following suggestions, particularly if you desire ultimately to return to clinical medicine:

1. Consider the field of medicine you would like eventually to follow and, after discussing the matter with your supervisor, approach the relevant clinical departmental head with an offer of your clinical services for a prescribed, fixed portion of the week. Some clinically attuned supervisors will do this for you. Be aware that it is unlikely you will be remunerated for this time.

2. Outpatient and operating sessions are valuable as they are well-circumscribed entities consistent with reliable planning of the rest of the week's research.

3. Try to make these clinical commitments relevant to your future interests or, best of all, to your current research. For example, if your laboratory project is a study of the effects of growth hormone on the healing of burns, a session a week assisting the plastic surgery team in theatre for a burns dressing and grafting list would be ideal. If your thesis is an electron microscopic investigation of lymphomas, you might consider attending the haematological or lymphoma outpatient clinic or ward round.

4. Obtain a contract, even if only an honorary one, from your employing body in the hospital setting out a specified number of clinical hours per week. In the UK at present, all honorary clinical (even part-time) jobs within the National Health Service are recognized as being full-time in terms of salary scales. For example, if you do three years as a part-time honorary Speciality Registrar during your research years, when you return to a full-time position, you will be paid as a fourth-year Speciality Registrar.

5. Similarly, your employer may pay Legal Medical Defence subscriptions.

6. Weekly Grand Rounds and clinical meetings are also invaluable for keeping in touch.

On the other hand, you should consider the following precautions:

1. Never get a 'bleep'/pager. One of the positive aspects of a period of research that you should enjoy is that you are a free agent. A pager by its very nature is a mental and emotional tie to a service, usually a hospital. It means people can contact you easily and at inconvenient times; for instance, during the middle of an intricate experiment.
2. Never be 'on call'. While on call you are responsible to patients and doctors. Although your periods of duty may be quiet, there will always be the potential for a distracting challenge at an inconvenient moment.
3. Be fastidiously firm with approaches from well-meaning people with requests for your services. Once you open the door to these demands, more and more approaches will flood in. Remember that your primary objective is to do your research and not to cover the hospital in case of clinical emergencies. If you maintain this firm line, your niche in the community will soon become established and respected.
4. Do not allow clinical obligations to take more than one day per week.

Extracurricular activities

Productivity of work towards a thesis increases with the time devoted to it. However, beyond a certain point, one tends to become less productive. Accordingly, include a variety of leisure activities while pursuing your research project to postpone this fall in productivity. In any case, some time taken well away from your research is necessary and beneficial. Extracurricular activities, whether they are sport, music, family, or a hobby, are good ways to achieve such a break and they positively influence morale, concentration and productivity. They also act as a 'buffer' for the times of minor mishap, disappointment and disaster that are inevitably associated with research.

Needless to say, there is a fine line between the beneficial and deleterious effects of extracurricular activities. Too much time and energy spent on other activities will detract from your research efforts.

Fitting in postgraduate medical examinations

Professional medical examinations, including the primary examinations of the Royal College of Physicians (MRCP) and Royal College of Surgeons (MRCS), those corresponding to other specialities, and the United States Medical Licensing Examination (USMLE: an examination necessary for working as a doctor in the US) are best completed early in one's postgraduate medical career. They require considerable study, and are best attempted during quiet jobs orientated toward the examination. In some cases, the early part of a period in research provides this opportunity. It is important to check the requirements and dates of these examinations with the relevant College or Board to determine if you can fit preparations for such examinations into your programme. However, consider 'compartmentalizing' these activities. In other words, devote a significant focused period of time to the relevant examinations and get them out of the way before embarking on research. The research can then be 'compartmentalized' without the distraction of examinations or clinical work.

Getting started with clinical research

Unless you are joining a group working on an existing clinical trial or are analysing data from an earlier study, much of the early research period with clinical research will be spent planning your project and gaining approval to carry it out. In contrast to laboratory research where a hypothesis is proven or refuted through a series of short, linked experiments, clinical research often involves one or more longer studies. The planning phase therefore takes substantially longer and, in addition to formulating a question and developing a detailed study protocol, requires gaining ethical and local clinical approval. This process can take a significant period of time and is almost always iterative, with multiple revisions and changes in the study design. To avoid unnecessary delays, it is worth seeking advice about the sample size requirements, costs and acceptance from clinicians and statisticians early in the process.

Getting started at the bench

Much of 'getting started' involves combining the ideas for research with the available facilities, time and literature to produce experimental results.

Early 'hands on' in the laboratory is essential. Initially, do not be too concerned about experimental design or what you are testing. Simply set yourself (or have your supervisor set you) a very simple problem in order to familiarize yourself with a particular laboratory technique or a group of related techniques that will be fundamental to your research. Once that technique is mastered, move to the next in the sequence, all the while contemplating how you could use these techniques to test an interesting hypothesis, and/ or how you can improve the technique. Once you know roughly what works, how easy or difficult it is, and how long it takes, you can set yourself simple hypotheses to test, and plan some experiments. While doing this, continue to review the literature at times when you are unable to be by the bench.

Too many research students, however, tend to devote too much attention to the literature. It is much easier to go into the library and read some journals than it is to walk into an unfamiliar laboratory and begin an experiment. You could spend forever reviewing the literature; it is important, but stifling. Obsessive reading fosters a negative frame of mind and makes you think about what you cannot do, not what you can do.

Choosing laboratory techniques

Much time in the early stages of pursuing research is spent assessing the facilities and techniques that are available to you.

A *useful technique* is one that:

1. is regularly performed in your laboratory,
2. is reproducible,
3. has controls already in existence,
4. is easy to set up,
5. produces rapid results that you can assess, and
6. produces simple and unambiguous results.

A *less useful technique* is likely to have one or more of these disadvantages:

1. untried,
2. not reproducible,
3. difficult to perform and expensive in money and time,
4. takes long to produce results (months/years), and
5. produces ambiguous results.

A supervisor experienced in the techniques that you employ and the ways of approaching your problem is particularly helpful. You will still have a feeling of independence if your project is close enough to your supervisor's own work to interest him, but distant enough so that you are pursuing an interest of your own.

Planning experiments

When planning your experiments consider the following suggestions:

1. *Don't be too ambitious:* the first experiment, carefully done and with small numbers, often works. It is when you complicate the experimental design with extra groups, variables and numbers that it falls apart and the data become impossible to interpret!

2. *Analyse results as you* go *along:* proper and prompt analysis, although initially apparently time-consuming, is ultimately more efficient as it allows the researcher to plan more effective subsequent experiments.

3. *Avoid heroics:* start with simple experiments that work and gradually progress upwards. Allow time for unforeseen but inevitable disasters (e.g. broken equipment, unavailable chemicals).

4. *Number of projects:* have more than one activity running at any given time. Most experiments entail periods of waiting, and it is useful to 'dovetail' several of these together in order to use your time most effectively, but not to the point where you end up with distractions, confusion and mistakes.

5. *Weekly routine:* consider establishing a weekly routine. For instance, you might carry out a planned experiment early in the week or early in the day. Analyse the previous week's results midweek, and prepare for next week's activities late week. Have set days and times for your clinical and extracurricular activities.

6. *Label your samples, containers and computer disks:* identify all materials with your name, the date of purchase and/or purpose, preferably in a colour specific to you. Keep them together in the refrigerator, freezer or shelf, so that they can be found and identified unambiguously when in a hurry.

Keeping careful notes

Above all, keep careful notes of procedures and results in your laboratory notebook. A hard-backed, lined exercise book is an essential aid to planning, carrying out and analysing your experiments.

1. *Date* each day's work.
2. Write the *aim* of the experiment.
3. *Materials:* record the model, manufacturer and code number of equipment and sources of chemicals used the first time you

use a new piece of equipment or chemical. This procedure saves much time and energy later on.

4. *Methods:* include full notes and related citations for all your procedures.

5. Make a note when you alter a standard procedure, with the date and the exact details of the alteration. Similarly, do likewise should you subsequently return to the original method.

6. Always write or stick the *results* directly into the book.

7. *Analysis:* when something goes wrong (e.g. mixing-up tubes, adding the wrong chemical) write it in. Something that appears obvious at the time will be forgotten months or years later.

8. Number the pages and set up an *index* at the back of your book (or on computer) so that results and procedures can be found easily.

Analysing results

The 'results' phase of any period of research is the most rewarding. However, except in those clinical studies that have defined end-points, it often arrives gradually and insidiously as your methods and thoughts develop and crystallize. It may only be on reflection that you appreciate how much has been achieved. The priority at this stage is to keep up the momentum. You will by now hopefully have established patterns and methods of using your time. Stick to them and 'crunch out' the results! Don't forget the importance of analysing your results early and as you go along though. It is not appropriate to place undigested records of your findings in a pile to be sifted through whilst you are writing up months or even years hence.

It is also worth checking the university regulations governing the format of illustrations and their preparation near the start of your project. You should then make a conscious decision at an early stage as to how you will label your graphs, what units you will use and how you want to express them. Make a note of this style and stick to it.

Once a reasonable set of results are to hand, you may wish to present them to your colleagues and peers for comments and criticism. Indeed, many programmes require postgraduate students to present their findings at departmental seminars. You may be encouraged by your supervisor to go further and display your work to a wider view, possibly through presentation at a meeting, verbally, by poster, or both, or by submission of a paper for publication (see Chapter 11).

Consulting a statistician

It is beyond the scope of this book to discuss statistical analysis of data in any great detail. Nearly all medical researchers have some acquaintance with basic statistics, but there is no easy way to acquire insight into all the important statistical concepts and principles. Attendance at a course if available in your University or department will remind you of the basic principles that you need to bear in mind when designing and interpreting experiments. However, statistics is not as 'cut and dried' a subject as you might expect. Good statistical analysis requires common sense and judgement, as well as a repertoire of formal techniques. It is often not possible to prescribe one statistical method for all the data analysis bearing upon a given problem.

It is therefore advisable to consult a statistician at an *early* stage while planning your experiments, particularly if your project requires analysis of lots of figures. Doing this will result in additional advantages:

1. You begin a professional relationship with the expert which will continue and develop as the project unfolds.
2. The statistician can advise you on the sample sizes you are likely to require to make the experiment or study statistically

valid. Mistakes in experimental design often cannot be rectified retrospectively when analysing data.

3. The statistician may suggest a method of data collection that will make statistical analysis simpler.

4. The statistician will direct you to an appropriate choice of statistical method, and may arrange access to the appropriate statistical software for later analysis.

5. You will have greater confidence in your statistical methods if your examiners or referees criticize them.

Planning ahead

By now one would hope that you are up and running, and that you have found some methods that work and some hypotheses to test. These are heady days, for you feel you are getting a grip on the 'tools of science' and it is now a matter of putting them into practice. Before getting too carried away, you might consider some cautionary words of advice that may save time and problems later:

1. *Set yourself flow charts* to map out how you have progressed and where you are heading.

2. *Continually assess.* Make sure you understand the results you are getting. If not why not? Write your thoughts down. Don't necessarily dismiss odd or 'quirky' results. They may end up being the most interesting.

3. *Think ahead.* Plan for unforeseen circumstances, and for foreseen delays. For example, apply for your animal procedures licence well in advance while working out the details of your experiment. Order required equipment and chemicals well before you actually need them. By the time these arrive, you may be ready to proceed.

4. *Be flexible.* Although planning is laudable, you should never be so rigid that you cannot follow a new avenue or drop an unrewarding one.

Writing research reports

Many faculty boards, funding bodies and supervisors ask for periodic progress reports from research students on their work. While this may seem annoying and constricting while you are in full experimental flight, they do have several important functions. These include:

- focusing your mind on which hypotheses you are testing and how you are testing them;
- giving you practice at scientific writing; and
- providing a useful store of organized information to be used when you come to write up your thesis.

Following the literature

An important, indeed vital, part of your research is the review of previous publications in your field of study and in its related topics. Such a literature review has a number of essential functions:

1. It provides you with an idea of the current state of knowledge in the field and enables you to identify possible gaps where further work might be of value.
2. It details the research techniques employed in the study.
3. It will form an important part of two portions of any scientific writing, the Introduction and the Discussion (see Chapter 10).

As already mentioned, however, do not try to carry out an exhaustive literature search before you start your own experimental investigations. First of all, this will depress you to see just how much is already known about your topic and, secondly, following up the resulting bibliography will take up such a horrendous amount of time that your available period of research will be spent mainly in the library! Rather, a preliminary review is often better based on selected papers and/or monographs which your supervisor will provide. They should be enough to get you started with the aims of the project and details of the techniques that you will be using. Most, if not all, of these should be well known to your supervisor and other members of the laboratory staff.

Reviewing the literature will continue all through your research period. Appropriately directed reading will draw your attention to fresh opportunities for experimental study of which you might not otherwise have been aware. Conversely, areas which you might otherwise have pursued relentlessly may turn out to be of marginal interest or already intensively studied, not justifying a time-consuming investigation. You should continue to follow developments in the literature after submitting your thesis while awaiting your oral examination, even if this involves a wait of several months. It would be unfortunate if you missed an important review article or publication in a well-read journal which appeared just a few weeks before your viva and which your examiners had read or, worse still, which one of them had actually written!

At present there are more than 10 000 medical journals published annually, and each year the number increases. Fortunately, there are a number of online databases that allow you to search by author, title, keyword, date, journal, etc., or a combination. Some also allow you to sign up for alerts so that you are sent e-mails with details of recently published articles in your area of interest. Some of the most comprehensive sites include:

- *MEDLINE* (Medical Literature Analysis and Retrieval System Online) – the US National Library of Medicine's premier bibliographic database that contains over 16 million references to journal articles in life sciences with a concentration on biomedicine. A distinctive feature of MEDLINE is that the records are indexed with NLM's Medical Subject Headings (MeSH) enabling more accurate searching. It is the major component of PubMed and can also be accessed via the NLM Gateway.
- *PubMed* (www.pubmed.gov) – a freely accessible online database of biomedical journal citations and abstracts compiled by the US National Library of Medicine. It includes all articles indexed for MEDLINE (approximately 5200 journals published in the US and more than 80 other countries) as well as citations to articles

before they are indexed for MEDLINE, that precede the date that a journal was selected for MEDLINE indexing and that are out-of-scope. It features links to many sites providing full text articles and other related resources, and allows the reader to store collections of citations and save and automatically update searches.

- *The NLM Gateway* (http://gateway.nlm.nih.gov) – a 'one-stop shop' providing a single interface online that searches in multiple retrieval systems, including MEDLINE/PubMed, ClinicalTrials.gov and OMIM.
- *The Cochrane Library* (www.thecochranelibrary.com) – consists of a range of Cochrane reviews, other systematic reviews, clinical trials, methods studies, technological assessments and economic evaluations which are particularly relevant to evidence-based clinical practice.
- *Scopus* (www.info.scopus.com) – the largest abstract and citation database of research literature and quality web sources containing 36 million records from over 16 000 peer-reviewed journals and 386 million quality web sources, including 22 million patents. As well as offering facilities to search for articles, this site also has useful details on individual authors, including a summary of their published work and the number of times their articles have been cited by other articles. It requires an institutional subscription.
- *Embase* – a biomedical database covering around 3500 journals from 110 countries, with particular strengths in the fields of drug research, pharmacology and toxicology.
- *Biomed Central* (www.biomedcentral.com) – an independent publishing house providing immediate open access to 196 peer-reviewed biomedical research journals.
- *ClinicalTrials.gov* (http://clinicaltrials.gov) – a registry of clinical trials conducted in the US and around the world.
- *OMIM* (www.ncbi.nlm.nih.gov/omim/) – a database of human genes and genetic phenotypes containing information on all Mendelian disorders and over 12 000 genes.

Medical libraries are also an important and useful resource. They differ greatly between themselves in organization, but perhaps the single most important thing to do is to know your own library and particularly its staff. Most librarians are used to being asked for advice on how to perform searches and larger University libraries will also offer courses on web-based journal searching. When starting a literature search:

- don't expect to be able to do the whole search in one line;
- don't expect your first attempt to get all the articles you need; and
- try to think of alternative ways of searching around your topic.

Critically appraising the literature

As well as finding the relevant literature, it is important to appraise it critically. In general this involves thinking about the following questions as you read any paper:

1. Are the results of the study valid?
2. What are the results?
3. Will the results help locally?

A number of checklists have been developed to help with this. Details of these can be found at the Department of Health Public Health Resource Unit website (www.phru.nhs.uk). It is important, however, not to rely solely on checklists. They are a useful guide (particularly as an aide-memoire), but they are not a substitute for thinking.

Compiling references

During the course of your research you will accumulate a large number of references. As an increasing number are now available online, it is likely that you will store most of these on computer. For articles whose full text is not available online, it is worth photocopying them and filing them in some form of order for future reference, or performing the electronic equivalent. There are a number of bibliographical software programmes designed to store, collate and insert references into documents which are invaluable. It is worth starting to use one of these programmes early in your research as it will save time later. A useful comparison of the various different programmes is available at: http:// en.wikipedia.org/wiki/Comparison_of_reference_management_ software. The most commonly used in medical research are *Endnote*, *Reference Manager* and *Procite*. Some universities supply this software at no charge.

Most of these programmes will allow you to select the output style of references in documents and will have pre-saved formats for many journals. Most universities will allow you to choose the format of references in your thesis, but probably the most popular way is the Harvard citation system, which gives author and year of publication in the text, and the full reference in the reference list. In this system:

1. In the text, authors' surnames are given in the order in which they appear in the research paper, followed by the date in brackets [e.g. Smith, Martin & Jones (1989)]. In the reference list, authors' initials must also be given, and the full reference details.

2. If there are more than three authors, then in the text the first author's name is given followed by '*et al.*' [e.g. 'The validity of the method was investigated by Smith *et al.* (1989) …'], but all the authors are named in full in the reference list. [NB This is why while making notes of your references you should keep a record of all the authors. Furthermore, some journals ask for the list of authors in full, and it is always easier to delete details than to add them.]

3. If the same authors published more than one paper in the same year, and these works are cited in the text, then the date is suffixed with 'a' or 'b', etc.

4. If the article is a chapter in a book, name the article, and its authors, as well as the title, publisher and the editor of the book.

Summary

- Getting started can be a difficult transition from clinical practice and involves a number of important steps.
- Much of 'getting started' involves choosing techniques and carefully planning experiments.
- Keep meticulous records.
- Maintain your clinical connections – but not at the expense or detriment of your research work.
- Review publications in your field and compile research references as you proceed.

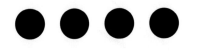

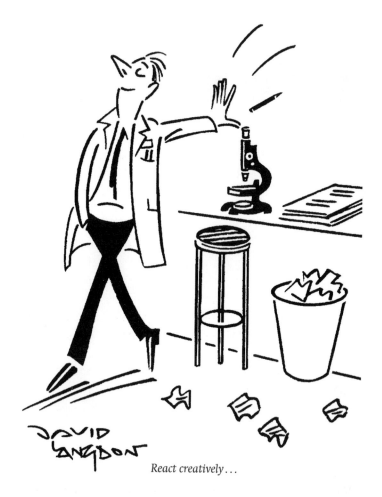

React creatively . . .

8

Overcoming frustration

Inevitably the heady days of early successes, new techniques and new equipment come to a resounding end when the inherent weakness of the procedure, equipment, hypothesis, approach, or even the problem you have set yourself become manifest. Setbacks and failures in research are inevitable. Being aware of this, and realistic about it, will help you to cope. It is important not to take such events too seriously, but to treat them in an analytical, almost detached fashion, as yet further problems to solve.

In addition, it is important to be clear that not obtaining positive results, or the findings that you expected, need not invariably be identified with failure. Disproving a particular point conclusively can be as constructive and scientific an outcome as proving a hypothesis. Initial negative results may provide a warning about the appropriateness or validity of the hypothesis being explored. However, it is genuinely disheartening when experiments do not seem to work at all and fail to give any interpretable results. Individuals vary a great deal in the way they react to such obstacles. Here are some alternatives, whose applicability would vary with the particular situation at hand.

Repeat the same procedure
- Do this when you think the procedure you have adopted is fundamentally sound, but that you may have performed it with less skill than you might have wished, or feel you require further practice in performing the procedure itself.

- This course of action is desirable provided that you re-examine the situation and assess the problem before you repeat.
- This course of action is inappropriate if it involves repeated uncritical attempts without thinking about the reasons for the lack of success.

Alter the procedure or method of attack

- Try this if your original response was tentative, and you can reinterpret the problem and attempt a new approach.
- This course of action is appropriate if the altered tactics are based on a careful analysis of the problem and the previous method or attack is also given due assessment and criticism.
- This approach is undesirable if the new method is adopted thoughtlessly.

Modify your goal

- Try this if an alternative goal is available, or if you no longer expect the original goal to be attainable. Alternatively, you may feel the original goal was not a high priority in your overall project, or that alternative approaches might be tried to complete it.
- This decision is desirable if:
  - the new goal satisfies the same needs as the original one;
  - the new goal leads to learning something useful;
  - the original goal is unimportant or not feasible.
- This action is undesirable if:
  - the substitute goal is also unrealistic;
  - you are retreating when reasonable further effort will result in success;
  - the substitute goal actually unbalances the overall plan of your project.

Give up the procedure or goal

- You are likely to select this course of action if you do not expect to succeed in your original goal, or if you think the goal is unimportant, or the means to achieve it are too difficult.

- An alternative is to return to the problem later in the project.
- This course of action is undesirable if reasonable further effort will, in fact, ensure success.

Quite clearly, the appropriate course of action varies with circumstances, and good judgement is necessary. If you continually fail to obtain meaningful results or the methods are still not working, you must seriously consider changing direction, and this may involve the research project, laboratory or even supervisor. In situations like this, your supervisor will be particularly helpful. He will have more experience and a better intuitive 'feel' of what is or is not going to work. You can also help yourself by keeping a well-annotated and full practical book that fully documents your experimental procedures, conditions and outcomes. This is invaluable when trouble-shooting unexpected or unsuccessful experimental outcomes. Finally, altering one's goal should not necessarily be seen as merely an 'easy way out'. Goals should remain flexible, since often new and more interesting goals will present themselves as work progresses.

Summary
- Setbacks in research are almost inevitable.
- Negative findings can be as important as positive ones.
- Remain flexible and be prepared to alter your approach.

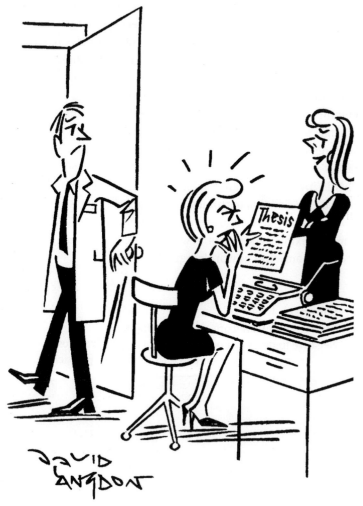

'Heavens! You don't expect intelligible *writing*
from doctors . . .'

9

Writing scientifically

How you structure your writing and express your ideas profoundly influences your readers' and, more importantly, your examiner's impression and understanding of your work. A small number of talented, experienced and much practised writers are able to write quickly and fluently, but most of us require considerable effort to make our writings acceptable. The brief remarks in this section cover the important steps to be taken when writing, and may provide some help on how to compose scientific prose and indicate some of the reasons why a given piece of scientific writing may be unsatisfactory. However, they cannot replace more substantial volumes on the use of English, to which the reader must refer if he or she wants more definitive details.

Decide what to say

The first step in writing is to be absolutely clear as to what you want to say. The best English in the world will not compensate for a writer with nothing to report. Note down in a rough, not necessarily logical, fashion a list of the points you wish to make. They can then be ordered later, or in the course of writing.

Organize what you wish to say

Determine how your writing needs to be organized. This will vary depending on whether you are writing a progress report, a research paper or your thesis. Broadly speaking, though, most scientific writing follows the IMRaD style (Introduction, Methods, Results and Discussion) and includes the following sections.

1. Abstract or summary.
2. Introduction.
3. Materials and methods.
4. Results.
5. Discussion.
6. Bibliography or references.

Think about the order of writing

Although the above will be the final order of your thesis or paper, consider completing their actual writing or drafting in a different order. The Methods section is usually straightforward and best done during or soon after completing the study. The Results is the most important section for the reader and time is well spent organizing this section early. It may seem counterintuitive, but the Introduction section is often easier to write after you have your results, as you can focus on what is relevant to your study and how best to 'whet' the appetite of your reader. If you write your introduction first you are likely to include a lot of information with little relevance to your final study.

Abstract or summary

This provides a brief and succinct summary of the work performed and is usually controlled by word limit and format stipulated by the journal or required in the thesis you are writing. It is imperative to follow these requirements. For some reports you will be required to write this in a structured format, but even in the absence of a defined format, it should have a clear paragraphed layout. In the absence of a stipulated word limit, online abstracts for research papers are often truncated at 250 words, so this is a good length to aim for. Remember that it is the first thing that people will read. Much therefore depends on it and the greatest care should be taken in its preparation. It is the shortest part of your paper, report or thesis, but it is probably the most important! By all means have a rough draft of your summary produced at an early stage. However, in practice it is usually the last section to be written definitively.

For original research articles, whether the abstract is required to be structured or not, you should include the following:

1. A few lines stating the overall aims of the work and the early findings that prompted the project.
2. A brief passage on the methods and procedures employed, referring particularly to the species used and experimental controls.
3. One or more sentences outlining the principal experimental findings, in logical sequence (not necessarily described in the chronological order in which they were actually obtained).
4. A summary of the principal conclusions, followed by some reference to their implications.

For structured abstracts, the headings will vary depending on the type of study you are writing up and the journal you are submitting to. For example, the following subheadings are required by the *British Journal of Medicine*:

[1] For standard original clinical research articles:

1. Objectives – a statement of the main aim of the study and the major hypothesis tested or research question posed.
2. Design – including factors such as randomization, blinding, placebo control, case control, crossover, criterion standards for diagnostic tests, etc.
3. Setting – include the level of care, e.g. primary, secondary; number of participating centres.
4. Participants – numbers entering and completing the study, sex and ethnic group if appropriate, including clear definitions of how selected, entry and exclusion criteria.

5. Interventions – details of what, how, when and for how long.
6. Main outcome measures – those planned in the protocol and those finally measured.
7. Results – main results with 95% confidence intervals and, where appropriate, the exact level of statistical significance and the number needed to treat/harm.
8. Conclusions – primary conclusions and their implications, suggesting areas for further research if appropriate.
9. Trial registration – registry and number for clinical trials.

[2] For meta-analyses and systematic reviews:

1. Objective – what the review set out to determine.
2. Design – type of meta-analysis, systematic review.
3. Data sources – where included studies were retrieved from.
4. Review methods – inclusion and exclusion criteria.
5. Results – main findings with 95% confidence intervals.
6. Conclusions – primary conclusions and their implications.

[3] For Qualitative research articles:

1. Objective.
2. Design.
3. Participants.
4. Setting.
5. Results.
6. Conclusions.

Introduction

The Introduction provides a concise account of the work of previous investigators in the general field of your research and justifies the importance of your study.

As mentioned above, it is worth considering writing this section last and it is often helpful to include the following:

1. A brief historical setting: what happened at the beginning, how ideas developed, how new techniques helped, pointing

out existing gaps in understanding (to be filled in, of course, by your own work!).

2. A thorough coverage of the set of papers immediately leading up to the work you have done.
3. An introduction to your research justifying why you chose this particular question and its importance to the general field.
4. Some authors provide a brief summary of their principal findings or their implications.

Methods

The Methods section provides details of how your experiments or procedures were performed and results analysed. For clinical studies, it must include full details of how participants were selected, including entry and exclusion criteria, and details of the interventions undertaken. It should provide sufficient detail both to enable your findings to be repeated on future occasion and to make clear the appropriateness of your procedures and your adequate provision of experimental controls. You should therefore aim to make your Methods section:

1. Full and explicit: previously described methods need not be reproduced in detail, but appropriate reference to the original, and often a brief resumé, should be included.
2. Reproducible: there should be enough detail for your experiments to be repeated on a future occasion. Diagrams of your apparatus can be useful.
3. Concise: within the above limitations, you should aim to present the methods as clearly and concisely as possible.

The name and address of the manufacturer of any instruments used for measurements should be given along with a catalogue number or instrument identification (e.g. Model DG2A; Digitimer, Welwyn Garden City, UK). In the case of solutions for laboratory use, the methods of preparation and precise concentration should be stated and the name and address of the supplier for non-standard constituents included.

All statistical methods should be identified. They can be mentioned after describing the relevant method or in a separate section. When several statistical techniques are used, it should be absolutely clear which method was used and where. Very common techniques, such as t-tests, simple χ^2 tests, analysis of variance, Wilcoxon and Mann–Whitney tests, correlation and linear regression, do not need to be described in detail. Variants of particular methods, such as paired and unpaired t-tests, should be identified unambiguously. More complex methods do require explanation, and precise references should be given for unusual methods. It may be helpful to comment briefly on why a particular method of analysis was used, especially if a more familiar approach was available. Where appropriate, you should name the computer program or software package used. When doing so, the particular statistical methods employed should still be identified.

Results

When planning the Results section, it often helps first to decide upon, and even prepare, the illustrations, including graphs and tables, that you wish to include and the order in which you wish to present them. You should try to set out your results in a logical order, not necessarily in the chronological sequence in which you actually performed your experiments. Begin with those results that validated the experimental technique, or with the early, simplest and most straightforward results. If appropriate, a careful and systematic description of the data should follow. In general, variables which are important for the validity and subsequent interpretation of statistical analyses should be described in more detail. Follow with the confirmatory experimental results. Leave the more sophisticated or complicated results to the end.

Clarify and emphasize your controls. Deviations from the intended study design should be described. For example, in clinical trials it is important to enumerate withdrawals from treatment allocation, with reasons, if known. In surveys, where the response rate is of fundamental importance, it is valuable to give information on how the non-responders differed from those who took part.

Discussion

The Discussion section relates your work to the background of existing knowledge on the subject, and demonstrates how your results have advanced the field. For example, the hypothesis which arose from the research papers you reviewed in your Introduction may now have been proven or refuted, the clinical observations of previous workers confirmed and expanded, or your experimental observations may have shed light on that hypothesis. Think of it as an opportunity to persuade the reader that your research is important and will lead somewhere in the future.

Many workers begin by summarizing the techniques employed and their validity (if they are new), and the major findings. Although this seems repetitious, it helps you emphasize the major results, so facilitating your arguments to follow.

This will lead naturally to an immediate interpretation of your findings. Outline what your results mean, without extensive details of data analysis, but emphasize comparisons with the controls. You should include enough information and argument to convince the reader of your central message.

You will then wish to relate your results to other findings in a manner that will depend on the nature of your work and the history of the field. For example, your project may have been prompted by earlier findings suggesting an interesting line of study. If so, you need to summarize these earlier findings, what they suggested, and where your findings now lead. Alternatively, you may have sought to resolve apparent (or real) discrepancies between earlier findings. If so, you will want to discuss the extent to which your results resolve the controversy. Finally, you may have entered a little explored area about which hardly anything is known. You will then be presenting a set of novel phenomena, which you should lay out as clearly as possible, before proceeding to more speculative interpretations.

You may wish to conclude with a broader coverage of ideas and hypotheses arising from your results, and their relationship to your surveyed field as a whole.

It is clear from this that Discussion sections vary greatly between papers and between authors, and closely reflect both the particular experiments performed and the hypothesis at hand, and current thinking in the field. For this reason, they are often demanding to write, particularly when considering both unexpected results and explaining possible errors. Perhaps a useful checklist is to ensure that the Discussion has made established the following major assertions:

1. That the work has made significant and coherent findings.
2. That the experiments were performed correctly and appropriately controlled, using suitable methodology.
3. That the findings were important to the subject at hand.
4. That the outcomes of the paper are likely to lead on to further developments in the subject.

Appendices

Appendices can be useful for material whose inclusion in the main body of the paper would disrupt the flow of text. This might include epidemiological questionnaires, mathematical derivations, details of statistical tests, clinical details of patients and computer programs.

Plan your writing

Any reasoned argument requires a logical sequence. Consequently, before writing any section, you should order your thoughts to create a logical outline of your subject matter.

1. Break down each section of your planned work into shorter, manageable units.
2. Then think carefully about your order of presentation.
3. Draw up a list of subheadings and subdivisions, and organize them into a layout that you will use consistently.

Write quickly

Once you have prepared an outline, you can then work towards a first draft or each successive section in your plan by dictating or writing quickly. Leave spaces for the details. You can always look these up later. The priority at this stage is to keep up the flow and momentum of your thoughts. At a later date you can refine the text, fill in details, add extra thoughts, correct obvious errors and make sure that your English is appropriate.

Scientific English

Your scientific prose should next undergo a process of evolution and reorganization, with the text being shortened where redundant, expanded, clarified and corrected as necessary with each revision.

1. Make sure that your vocabulary is adequate for, and appropriate to, the subject matter being discussed. This entails being familiar with and understanding the relevant terminology, and making certain that your meaning is clear. Every individual uses different sets of words in different aspects of his or her everyday life. However, in scientific writing, these vocabularies may be inappropriate, or imply a different meaning. Using colloquialisms and stock phrases leads to inaccuracies and misunderstanding, and conveys an impression of lack of care and thought. Select words that best convey your technical meaning, even if a simpler but less accurate word is available. However, subject to the above proviso, use short, clear, familiar words in preference to long unfamiliar ones.

2. Make sure the text is grammatically correct. Sentences should be generally short, well constructed and not depart from accepted or appropriate usage.

3. Check that transitions between sentences are smooth and logical. They may mislead the reader if they are too abrupt or misleadingly connected.

4. Make sure the sequence of the argument follows a logical order.

5. Make sure the passage is not written at a level of abstraction inappropriate for the reader.

6. Avoid 'I', 'me' and 'we'.

7. Use past tense as much as possible, e.g. 'the serum was diluted with PBS' rather than 'we mix the serum with PBS'.

Re-reading and re-drafting

All drafts, however well planned, demand careful re-reading and correction. After completing the initial version, leave it aside for a few days before you return to it for further work. Your colleagues and supervisor might very helpfully read through and comment on your text and this editing process may involve a number of exchanges backwards and forwards with your supervisor. As you approach the final revisions of your text, it is helpful systematically to review the overall content, then the individual paragraphs, sentences and words, as follows:

1. Content.
   Does the text depart from the main point being made in each section?
   Is there padding and irrelevance?
   Could the meaning be made clearer with further examples and illustrations?

2. Paragraphs.
   Does each paragraph form a natural unit?
   Is the transition from one idea or topic illogical or too abrupt?

Are some topics discussed out of context or left hanging in the air?

3. Sentences.

Are any sentences too long or involved?

Are any sentences unclear?

Are there any pronouns whose antecedents are ambiguous?

4. Words.

Are there vague, ill-defined words whose meaning is left undefined or unclear?

Are all terms employed with their accepted scientific meaning? For example 'significant' and 'significance' are words that are often used loosely in everyday writing. In a scientific text they should only be employed in their statistical sense, e.g. 'these findings were significant ($p<0.001$)'.

5. Tense and third person.

Is the text in the past tense and third person?

Summary

- Scientific writing is a learned art-form.
- The standard format is – Abstract, followed by Introduction, Methods, Results and Discussion – but this is not usually the order in which you will write up your thesis.
- Each section has a fairly standardized type of presentation.
- The Abstract (or Summary) is the first and the last thing your examiners will read – it is therefore the most important part of your thesis!

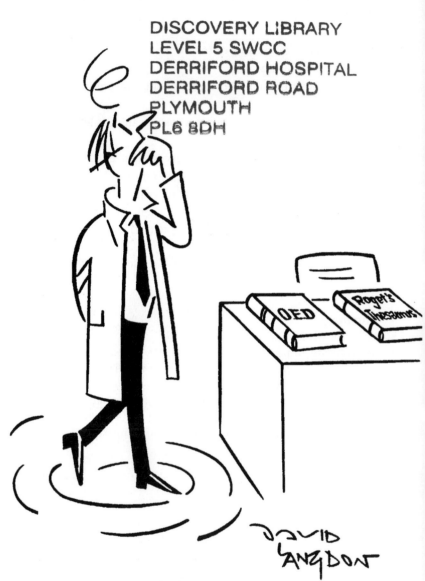

Decide what to say...

10
Publishing a paper

Deciding whether to write a paper

Hopefully at some point during your research you will acquire sufficient data to begin to publish your work in scientific or medical journals. In principle, the criterion for justifying preparing a paper is quite simple. You will have completed a substantial set of experiments that answer a scientific question in a number of important aspects, and you will have fully completed controls. Your findings then consequently come together to form a coherent body of knowledge that proves or disproves a particular hypothesis or provides information that is useful to the scientific community. However, judging the extent to which you have reached this point is a matter of experience. Your supervisor will be the best person to advise. In practical terms, having a number of submitted or published publications is a great reassurance as you plan your trajectory to finishing your research project. There are supervisors and research groups who encourage their students to write all their findings into research papers as their work proceeds. Completing a thesis is then greatly facilitated by simply assembling this work into a coherent whole!

Choosing when to write a paper

There are thus several advantages of publishing early on in your research period.

1. The exercise will concentrate your thoughts, reveal areas of inadequacy in your work and define areas for further testing. Thus the act of drafting a research paper itself facilitates your thinking about your work.
2. You will gain practice at scientific writing.
3. Most journals, whether they accept or reject your paper, will return copies of referees' comments. These usually contain important criticisms which range from grammatical and lettering mistakes, to omissions in your review of the literature and suggestions for further investigations. It is a great benefit to consider these criticisms in your own time, rather than in the heat of a thesis viva!
4. Many of the figures, tables and graphs you will prepare for submission for publication will be useful again in your thesis.

Under other circumstances you may choose to postpone writing up work for publications, particularly if your project is a monolithic one that is likely to finish with a single major work describing a large number of interrelated observations. This situation may occur if your work is part of a large multi-centre project, or involves a major clinical trial. Under these circumstances you will need to bear in mind that writing up will be a substantially more challenging exercise!

Choosing the journal

It can be difficult to decide on the particular journal to which you might submit your paper. Advice from your supervisor will be most helpful. Considerations include the following:

1. The quality of your paper, and the importance of its scientific contribution.
2. Your potential audience: whether you are aiming for a large medical and/or scientific audience, or a group of specialists.

Journals vary in a number of important respects:

1. Circulation: size of the readership.
2. Width of readership: international, national, regional or local.
3. Content and interest: scientifically or clinically orientated.
4. Breadth of interest: the degree of specialization of the journal.
5. Impact factor: the frequency with which articles from that journal are quoted.

Point 4 is exemplified below for medical journals.

Category	Example of journal
Broad scientific	*Nature*
Medicine in general	*British Medical Journal*
Speciality medical	*Journal of Bone and Joint Surgery*
Sub-speciality medical	*Journal of Hand Surgery*

A similar pattern exists for more scientifically orientated journals.

Category	Example of journal
Broad scientific	*Nature*
A field of science	*The Journal of Physiology*
Speciality in that field	*Biophysical Journal*
Sub-speciality	*Journal of Muscle Research and Cell Motility*

Writing a paper

The specific layout of a paper will vary with your specific field of research and the journal to which you decide to submit your article. Before starting to write, make sure you read the 'Instructions to authors' from the relevant journal carefully. These regulations are easily found on the internet, along with papers from recent issues of the journal to use as a model. These differences aside, the typical layout of a paper is:

1. Title page with the title of the paper, the names and addresses of all authors and the name and address of the author for correspondence.

2. Summary or abstract, including three to five keywords and in some cases a short running title up to 70 characters.
3. Introduction.
4. Methods.
5. Results.
6. Discussion.
7. Acknowledgements.
8. List of references.
9. Tables (including legends to tables).
10. Legends to figures with a new page for each legend.

Details of what to include in each of these sections is covered in detail in Chapter 9.

In addition to these sections, many clinical research papers also require supplemental files. Examples of these, with links to relevant websites, are given below, but the Equator Network (www.equator-network.org) also provides links to the main reporting guidelines and statements in one place.

- Clinical trial reports need to comply with the Consolidated Standards of Reporting Trials (CONSORT) and include a completed CONSORT checklist, the CONSORT-style structured abstract and the CONSORT flow diagram detailing the enrolment, intervention allocation, follow-up, and data analysis with number of subjects (see http://www.consort-statement.org).
- Systematic reviews require a completed QUORUM checklist and flow diagram (see www.equator-network.org).
- Meta-analyses of observational studies require a completed Meta-analysis of Observational studies in Epidemiology (MOOSE) checklist and flowchart (see Meta-analysis of observational studies in epidemiology: a consensus statement. *Journal of the American Medical Association* 2000, **283**(15), pp. 2008–12).
- Studies of diagnostic accuracy require a completed STARD checklist (see Towards complete and accurate reporting of studies of diagnostic accuracy: the STARD initiative. *Clinical Chemistry* 2003, **49**, pp. 11–6).
- Observational studies require a completed Strengthening The Reporting of OBservational studies in Epidemiology (STROBE)

checklist (see Strengthening the reporting of observational studies in epidemiology (STROBE) statement: guidelines for reporting observational studies. *British Medical Journal* 2007, **335**, pp. 806–08).

Preparing figures

The exact details will vary between different journals, but most now accept figures in the following formats:

1. Tagged image file format (Tiff) files – TIFF is the most universal and most widely supported format across all platforms. Files should ideally be at a resolution of 600 dpi. Note that you cannot get a high-quality tiff file by starting with a low-resolution one and changing the settings: you have to create a 600 dpi tiff in the first place. You can tell by magnifying; if the lettering looks sharp and crisp at high magnification the figure is fine, but if the lettering looks jagged the resolution at which the image was created was too low. To keep file size reasonable, the file should be compressed when prepared: when saving in the tiff file format look for a checkbox called LZW compression, and tick it.

2. PowerPoint® – figures can be submitted together in one PowerPoint® file for the editors later to convert into a PDF. In this conversion process the axes and scale bars will disappear if their 'weight' is 0 pt, so you should make the weight around 0.75 pt.

3. Portable document format (PDF) files – you will require high-resolution PDF files (the text and lines should be crisp and clear on-screen at 300 or 400%). This requires Adobe Acrobat Professional and the Press quality rather than Standard or Smallest File Size options in Conversion Settings.

4. Word processor files.

5. Encapsulated PostScript (EPS) files.

Most journals charge for colour figures, so think carefully about whether your figures really need to be in colour.

Preparing tables

In most journals, tables will be processed as text and therefore should not be submitted as figures or as 'pictures' inserted into a Word document, and should not be prepared in PowerPoint®. There are three recognized ways to prepare a table:

1. Use the Draw Table facility in Microsoft Word® or another word processor.
2. Separate columns of numbers separated by tab stops.
3. Prepare the table in Microsoft Excel® or another spreadsheet programme and then copy and paste the data into Microsoft Word®.

Submitting a paper

Most journals now accept submissions online through web-based programmes. It is possible to start submitting a paper and then save your work and return at a later time, but you will save yourself time if you have the following ready when you start:

1. The names, addresses and contact details for all the named authors.
2. A covering letter – this is optional for many journals, but if your paper follows on from previous work published in the journal or answers a specific question raised in a previous paper, then it is worth drawing attention to that here. You should also give details of any previous publications from the same study.
3. Names, addresses and contact details of potential referees.
4. The number of words (excluding references and figure legends), tables, black and white figures and colour figures in your paper.
5. The abstract.
6. A text document containing the title page, abstract, main body of text, references, tables and legends to figures.

7. Figures.
8. Any required supplemental files.

Once you have completed the online submission form and uploaded your text file and figures, the journal will convert them into one PDF file. This can take anything from 10 minutes to several hours. You will normally be notified by e-mail when the PDF is ready to view. You then need to go back to the submission site and check the PDF for potential conversion errors. You should pay particular attention to symbols, as some symbols inserted into Word files are often frustratingly converted to different symbols in PDF format. You also need to check that all of your references have been correctly identified by the journal. Once you are happy with the PDF file of your manuscript and the references, you need to confirm the submission of your paper.

Steps from submission to publication

If the journal decides to have the paper refereed, you may wait one to six months for a reply. On receiving referees' reports, the editor will do one of the following:

1. Reject your paper outright.
2. Accept the paper for publication, provided that you attend to the suggestions of the referees. These may range from minor omissions, to an extra experiment or two. When revising the paper in response to these requests, it is worthwhile to list each of the alterations you have made, corresponding to each of the referee's comments in your reply.
3. Accept the paper for publication without further alterations.

Once the final version of your paper has been accepted, the publisher may make minor adjustments and will set the text according to the printed style of the journal. Most publishers will send page proofs to you for final checking. You should particularly check the details of yourself and your fellow authors!

The time from submission to publication is often long (often a number of months). In general, weekly journals that have large international subscriptions (e.g. *Nature*, *The Lancet*) publish most promptly (sometimes in less than 3–6 months). Specialized journals that may only put out several issues a year are the slowest. To reduce this time lag, many journals have now introduced 'online before publication' facilities. You may also be offered the option, for a certain payment, for your work to be made 'open access'. This will have the advantage of making your work available to both the general public and the scientific community without subscription charge. Costs of this are often met by research funding agencies, for example the Wellcome Trust and British Heart Foundation.

Summary

- Your supervisor can advise whether to publish early or late in your research and help select the most appropriate journal.
- Before starting to write a paper, make sure you read the 'Instructions to authors' from the relevant journal carefully, as the precise format and presentation are standardized for each journal.
- Be prepared for it to take several months or longer, even after your paper has been accepted, before it is finally published.

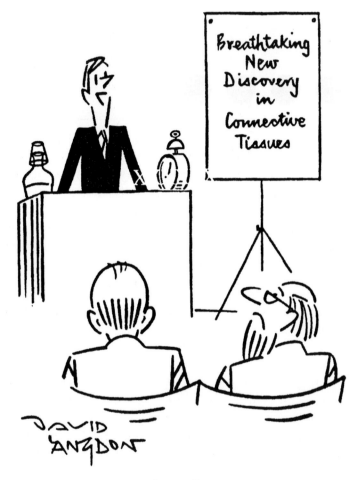

Presentation ...

11

Attending scientific meetings

Scientific meetings and conferences provide formal opportunities for researchers to get together and exchange information on a pre-defined subject or area of knowledge. They are also the ideal environment in which to develop your presentation skills. Application forms for clinical jobs are increasingly including sections for presentations, particularly at national and international audiences, and so a track record of presenting data has become an important part of career progression. Many of the larger conferences also publish the abstracts which can be beneficial for grant or other funding applications.

In general, the advantages of attending a meeting include:

1. making contact with, and gaining recognition from, other researchers in your field;
2. securing priority for your work by presenting it at a defined date;
3. getting practice in presenting work, and answering criticisms and questions (particularly useful for your approaching oral examination on your thesis); and
4. keeping up to date with progress in your field through contact with other participants and attending their presentations.

Choosing where to present

Within the general scope of scientific meetings, there is a hierarchy of forums at which you can display your work, ranging from informal discussion within your department to giving a paper at an international conference. These can be graded in ascending order as follows:

1. Seminar in your department.
2. Local meeting of a specialist society in your field, e.g. the London Connective Tissue Society Meeting.
3. National meeting of professional or academic societies, e.g. the British Connective Tissues Society.
4. International Conferences, covering a particular interest, e.g. International Symposium on Basement Membranes.
5. Major International Conferences, e.g. Gordon Conferences.

Each has its advantages and disadvantages. Departmental seminars are commonly informal and allow for more open discussion about your work and future direction. Local or regional meetings are often short and are useful for networking with local researchers. National meetings often last for several days and provide more scope for presentation and networking but most will require registration fees. International meetings carry the greatest prestige and many will publish abstracts, but travelling to exotic areas of the world can be expensive and time consuming.

Preparing oral presentations

Oral presentations typically range from 10 to 30 minutes with a period for questions at the end. There are many sources of advice for preparing oral presentations – here we simply list a few key points to consider:

1. Check that your topic being presented is within the scope of the meeting.
2. If possible, check in the advanced conference programme what the other presenters will be covering and to what depth, to avoid repetition and/or lack of background information.
3. Avoid complex animation sequences.

4. Rehearse your presentation against the clock in front of one, or preferably more, colleagues. There is usually a strict time limit on presentations and it is very frustrating to be stopped by the meeting's chairperson 30 seconds before you reach the climax of your talk.
5. Check whether you are required to send an electronic copy of your presentation prior to the meeting and always take a back-up copy with you.
6. Use presenter view in PowerPoint® to preview text for the next slide and allow you to see the speaker notes.

Preparing poster presentations

An increasing proportion of conferences now invite poster presentations as well as oral presentations and specific times are allocated at the meeting for presentation and discussion of posters. Some conferences ask for a one- or two-minute oral presentation of the poster to a small group or a few summary PowerPoint® slides, but most just require you to stand by your poster at the allocated times.

Most people choose to design posters using either Microsoft PowerPoint® or other design software. When designing a poster it is important to remember that it is an advertisement for your research. It is not simply a research paper wallpapered onto a board. The average interaction time for a poster is only a few minutes and most people will spend only a few minutes scanning the poster, so it is important that your poster attracts readers and highlights the important conclusions. Again, there are many sources of advice for preparing posters and, as with any design process, many elements are subjective, but here we have included a few hints to help produce an effective poster:

1. Make sure that you know the exact size and format for the poster session. If in doubt, contact the organizers.
2. If possible, use a landscape rather than a portrait format as this allows more content to be at eye level and avoids the risk of having all your conclusions at floor level.

3. Keep it simple. Simple messages are more memorable and are more likely to encourage people to stop and read your poster. Details can distract from the main point and can be added in person.

4. Try to present only one short central message. If you have a lot of material to present, or more than one message, submit two posters.

5. Use a column format so that the people reading it can start at one side and move to the other without having to go backwards and forwards. Consider adding numbering so that the order of presentation is explicit to the reader:

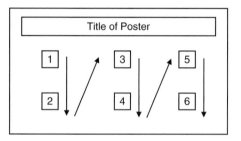

6. Keep text to a minimum – aim for about 30% text, 30% graphics and 40% empty space.

7. Remove all non-essential information from figures and make sure they are easily understandable and stand alone, separate from the text.

8. Try to avoid including material in the form of tables on posters since they generally require more attention and concentration from the reader.

9. Suggested minimum font sizes for the various parts of your poster are:
   a. Title: 85pt (depending on the length of the title).
   b. Sub-headings: 36pt
   c. Body text: 24pt
   d. Captions: 18pt

10. Make sure that you state a clear-cut conclusion.

Funding your visit

If the meeting is to be held in another city or overseas, you will naturally incur travel and accommodation expenses. Funding to help cover these expenses is variable and it is worth spending some time exploring the possible sources of funding available. A good place to start is your department, as these often have small funds available to support attendance at meetings. Some hospitals or universities may also contribute, so it is worth asking. A number of national societies also offer bursaries and, in some cases, if your work involves collaboration with a pharmaceutical or scientific instrument company, they may provide such funding.

Summary

- Attending and presenting at scientific meetings are important parts of your research training.
- Make use of the many sources of advice for preparing oral and poster presentations.
- It is worth spending some time exploring possible sources of funding for travel, registration and expenses at the meeting.

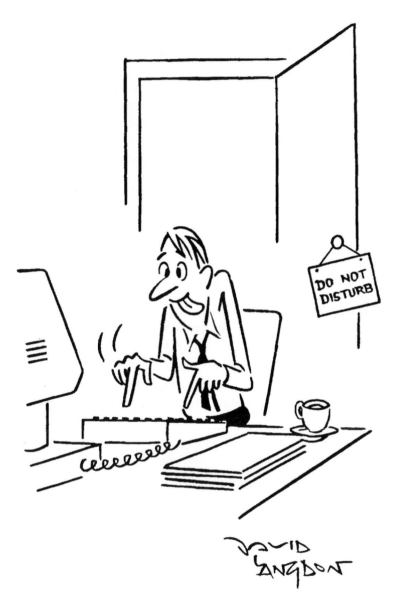

Writing the thesis...

⑫
Writing a thesis

Timing

Most students will reach a compromise between two extreme approaches to timing when it comes to writing up a thesis. You could start writing your dissertation only after completing all your experimental work, or could write a sequence of short accounts in the course of your project as you gather results and draw conclusions. Writing periodic progress reports and papers as circumscribed parts of your project become completed can form part of this process.

Writing continuously as you collect data has a number of advantages. It reduces the amount of pressure on you as you approach your thesis deadline, and encourages the good habit of reviewing and analysing data soon after they are obtained. The act of writing then becomes an integral part of your thinking about your data, dealing with inconsistencies, and identifying forgotten control experiments. These can then be rectified in the course of your continued laboratory work. In any case, writing as you go helps fill in periods where you are unable to do experiments; for example, when equipment is being serviced or repaired. Observing your dissertation as it gradually evolves, rather than anticipating the massive task of writing it, builds morale. Additionally, working some of your findings into publications will improve your chances of obtaining your next job, as then you will have something to show for your work. Finally, the time at which you decide to stop laboratory work and devote your time entirely to writing becomes less critical.

However, circumstances or inclination may lead you to leave any substantial writing to the end. Alternatively, you may persuade yourself that this course takes a smaller absolute amount of time or that you feel you can better keep your data in mind, as a whole, if you allocate large stretches of time entirely to writing.

Place

The timing of your writing up will in turn determine where you do it. If you draft your thesis in the course of your experimental work, it is likely that you will have time to write up your thesis while still in the laboratory. If you leave writing until you have completed all conceivable experiments, it is likely you will only get around to writing after you have left your laboratory. Most research students will take the most sensible choice of doing something in between.

If you get to do your writing up while still in your laboratory, you will be conveniently close to the equipment and chemicals you used and to advice from colleagues. Additionally, your supervisor may be close at hand to comment on your work as you progress. However, your colleagues still doing laboratory work may find your presence an obstruction; laboratories are often pushed for space, and other workers may also need the computer you are using. Finally, you may be more likely to be interrupted while in a busy laboratory.

Conversely there are some advantages to completing your writing away from the laboratory. You will be free from all distractions of a normal laboratory, and you may be able to look at your work more objectively. However, you then may not have some important sources of information to hand: you may realize while writing that you have forgotten your brand of foetal calf serum or the settings on your centrifuge. Additionally, depending on temperament, there are more distractions from composing when away from the laboratory.

A word of warning

A final possibility, which you should certainly try to avoid, is that you only get the opportunity to write up your thesis after you have left the laboratory, and you have already started your next employment. You will then combine the disadvantages of both the above options. You will not have the benefit of being near scientific advice and assistance, yet be readily distracted by colleagues in your new place of work, who may not be in the least interested in your previous work. You may also irritate your new senior colleagues or employer in being distracted by a commitment you still have to fulfil.

Furthermore, if you then take up an appointment which has a heavy clinical load, the quite considerable time you need to write up your thesis may just not be there. Finally, in what time there is available, you will find that you are tired, distracted, and all too often interrupted by clinical issues.

Winding up experimental work

It is very important, even while writing up, to allocate some time to return to the bench for some (usually minor) tidying up experiments; for example, those extra controls that the referee wants before your paper is published. One approach would be to keep one day or half a day a week working in the laboratory as you are writing, at least at the outset. You will then remain familiar with the layout of the laboratory and its facilities, and be in touch with any changes. A return to the laboratory after a prolonged absence can be very frustrating when all the chemicals have moved, and you have forgotten the minor intricacies of a particular method. The pressures of completing a thesis will amplify these frustrations.

When do you stop experimental work completely?

This is difficult to decide. There is a natural tendency for your supervisor to keep you hard at experiments; after all, to him your work is often part of a continuing project. On the other hand, students usually underestimate by at least 50% the time needed to perform particular tasks. This is especially the case for writing up theses. You will be surprised how long important processes such as reading and rewriting, printing out drafts, preparing illustrations and editing will take. Delays, of course, can be reduced by careful planning and setting up early on.

One rule of thumb is that if you have written and have had accepted two substantial papers (not just abstracts), or have sufficient data for two such papers that you expect will be accepted by reputable refereed journals, you have enough material for your MD or PhD thesis, and can turn from experimental work to writing up.

Planning your thesis

Completing a thesis is a formidable task. You should start planning and thinking about your thesis from the first day of your research project! It will fill your life for the duration of your research. In this connection, always have a notebook handy. You will be amazed at the times when insights about your research problem, or a minor flash of inspiration relevant to the dissertation, will occur. If you write down such thoughts, you can return to them later in a more objective frame of mind.

If you continually bear in mind the approach and organization you are trying to develop for your thesis, it will help you greatly in emerging with a clear picture of how you wish to organize your thesis at a relatively early stage. Generating an outline on your computer early on will encourage you to develop and improve it. To see the form of your thesis developing with time is encouraging and promotes work towards a more cohesive thesis.

Format of your thesis

As material, results and ideas develop, you will get a progressively better idea of the form your thesis will take. In addition, the nature of your thesis should be influenced by the following:

1. Studying the university regulations.

   Obtain the regulations for your degree in your university, and read and digest them, particularly governing preparation of theses and abstracts submitted for your particular degree.

2. Considering ways of organizing the material.

   In theory, you are relatively free to write your thesis as you like, provided that you follow university regulations. In practice, it is probably best to conform to tested ways of presenting work. There are two main possibilities, depending on the nature of your project. You could write your dissertation in a single coherent unit, organized into Introduction, Methods, Results and Discussion. Alternatively, you could write up separate components of your work in sequence, each in turn divided into separate Introduction, Methods, Results and Discussion, with a final common Discussion chapter which ties them all together. This latter format may be particularly appropriate if you have published a number of papers throughout your research. In most cases, though, your thesis will contain most or all of the following headings, varying slightly in order, reflecting different university regulations.

   - Title page and contents
   - Acknowledgements
   - Abstract
   - Introduction
   - Materials and methods
   - Results
   - Discussion
   - Future work and unanswered questions
   - Summary
   - Glossary and Appendices
   - Bibliography or Reference list
   - Publications

3. Inspecting past successful theses completed by others.

   It is helpful to examine as early as possible theses written in similar areas by your predecessors. These are often available in your university or departmental library. If you do this at an early stage, you will then be most influenced by appearance and least by content! You may also be able to locate, and pay particular attention to, your supervisor's own thesis. This exercise will illustrate to you ways to organize and lay out your material, and mistakes you may wish to avoid. Make notes on, or photocopy for your records, the appealing features of each thesis. You could use a particular thesis as an overall model, and aim to improve it by incorporating attractive features noted elsewhere.

4. Considering the length of different sections.
It is helpful to have a clear idea in your mind of the relative allocation of pages to the Introduction, Methods, Results and Discussion. The relative emphasis of each aspect will vary with project, and the amount and nature of your results. One approach might be to first decide upon your expected overall thesis length (giving due note to the regulations), then allocating 30–40% of the pages to the Results with as much as needed for the Methods. Divide the remaining pages roughly equally between the Introduction and Discussion. Then modify this basic scheme as needs become clearer as you do your writing up.

Writing the thesis

Actually starting to write can feel like a daunting process. To help this, the following is a frequently adopted order of writing:

1. Materials and methods.
2. Results.
3. Introduction.
4. Discussion.
5. Abstract.
6. Future work and unanswered questions.
7. Title page, contents and keywords.
8. Bibliography or reference list.

9. Glossary and Appendices.
10. Acknowledgements.

This sequence starts you off writing about simple hard facts, then subsequently progresses through observations, analysis and conjectures, to abstractions. General guidelines of what to include in the first five of these have already been discussed in Chapter 10. Sections specific to a thesis include the following.

Title page and contents

Most universities require you or your supervisor to propose a title early in your project. However, you will be able to adjust this at an appropriate stage, once you gather a clear indication of where your research is leading. Take care and advice over your final choice; the title should sum up the essence of your work in a short phrase. The title page should also include your name and address, the degree you are submitting the thesis for, and any other details that university regulations require.

If you are feeling particularly literate, or want to 'lighten up' a thesis, you might include a quotation. Make sure all quotations are accurate, correctly attributed and are directly relevant to the theme to which they refer. You should also include a clear contents list at the start of the thesis, and, in some cases, a list of illustrations.

Acknowledgements

A separate page should contain a list of acknowledgements, usually set out in paragraphs. If in doubt, choose to include rather than exclude individuals from your acknowledgements.

1. Thank your department and laboratory heads, at the very least, for access to facilities, and for other help, if this was given.
2. Your supervisor must be thanked.

3. You will wish to thank technicians and laboratory work-shops, the computer department, and any other members of the department who did much of the work assisting your passage.
4. There will probably be postdoctoral fellows and other colleagues who will have rendered invaluable aid and advice.
5. Acknowledge all individuals or agencies who lent you equipment.
6. Copyright permission should be included for direct reproductions from published material.
7. You need permission to cite unpublished data or personal communications in your thesis.
8. Be sure to acknowledge your funding body, and any title attached to your scholarship or grant.

Declarations

Most universities require you to include (and sign) a standard declaration within your thesis, concerning the extent to which the thesis was your original work, the extent to which some of the work was the result of collaborations, and if so, your contribution to it.

Future work and unanswered questions

No thesis is ever complete. It has been said that a good thesis will provide its author with enough work to occupy him or her for the rest of their professional life. One of the authors of this present book can vouch for this: he has continued to plod away in clinical and experimental studies based on his thesis on intra-abdominal adhesions for some 50 years – and still finds more questions which remain unanswered!

Unanswered questions and ideas for future work are sure to come to you. Even if they have not, they are certain to be in the mind of your examiner. Frequent questions asked in oral examinations include 'What further work arising from your thesis might you have in mind?', or 'Did you think of doing a further experiment using X instead of Y?' It is therefore well worth having a page or two in your thesis which discusses these questions, perhaps four to six of them, and you should devote perhaps one or two paragraphs to each.

Glossary

A glossary at the end, or sometimes a list at the beginning, of the thesis is sometimes used to define terms, abbreviations or unfamiliar concepts.

Publications

By the time your thesis is bound, you may already have one or more publications in journals, or abstracts in meetings where you presented your results. These should be quoted in the text, and listed in the bibliography. However, it is a good idea to insert the publications themselves into a flap placed inside the back cover of your thesis. If you have a paper in press but not yet published, it is still worth having a flap in place. The publication may appear during the delay which often intervenes between thesis submission and your oral examination. You can then bring the reprints with you to your viva, and give them to your examiners.

Successive draftings of the thesis

The first draft of a chapter or section should describe nearly all the experimental details, data and its analyses. References and cross-references to other parts of the thesis can be added later. At this stage your text will therefore be in rough form, but will contain most of the factual material you need to include. There will then be a good deal of moving, adding and deleting of text and checking minor points. Once this initial work is completed, you should read through the first draft to correct obvious mistakes.

In succeeding drafts you will make corrections, add further references to the text, adjust the English and vocabulary, and so work towards your final version. Depending on circumstances, it is helpful and instructive for you if your supervisor reads and comments at least on selected chapters as they are being written, preferably at an early stage, to ensure that you are on the right track. However, it is totally unrealistic and inconsiderate to expect your supervisor to drop all his commitments hurriedly to read a belatedly prepared effort given to him at short notice, just before a submission deadline. So start writing early to leave yourself and others a lot of time to manoeuvre.

Once all the components of the thesis are assembled, there follows a process of further work, usually pruning, by both yourself and your supervisor. Theses in their early stages are inevitably too long, so do not be too concerned if a great deal of material is subsequently omitted, particularly where there is repetition, or where you find material that is not relevant to the main thrust of the thesis.

Final checklist
The next step is to go through the whole thesis with a fine-tooth comb; a stage that may take up to a month!

A checklist might include:

Abbreviations. Are they really necessary?
      Are they explained clearly at the first occurrence?
      Can the reader find them quickly?
      Are they consistent?
      Have you considered including a list of these, together with their clarifications, at the beginning of the thesis for reference?

Format. Check the following for consistency of style and presentation:

- fonts,
- tables,
- figure legends,
- text headings,
- contents,
- references,
- appendices.

Numbering. Check that numbering sequences of the following are complete and consistent with references in the:

- tables,
- figures,
- text sections.

Correctness. Make a final check for accuracy in the:

- materials,
- methods,
- statistics,
- references,
- figures.

Language. Are certain expressions used too frequently?

Tenses. Check that these are correct throughout.

Plurals. For example, check data/datum, media/medium.

Spelling. Check for correctness and consistency.

Punctuation. Check for accuracy and reliability.

Layout. Does the text start a new page in the correct places? Is the page numbering correct?

Units. Make sure that all scientific units (kilograms, litres, etc.) are expressed using the correct abbreviations according to standard reference texts (e.g. *Quantities, units and symbols*, the Royal Society of London).

Figures. Make sure that the labelling on these is consistent with the text and legends. Check that you have used the same abbreviations, mathematical symbols, spellings and general style.

Summary

- Completing a thesis is a formidable task – you should start thinking about it from the first day of your research project.
- Depending on the nature of your research, you may plan to write your thesis only after completing all your experimental work or continuously as you collect data.
- Try to avoid having to write up your thesis after you have left research and returned to clinical practice.
- Before starting to write, check the University regulations and try to look at past successful theses completed by others.

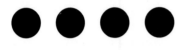

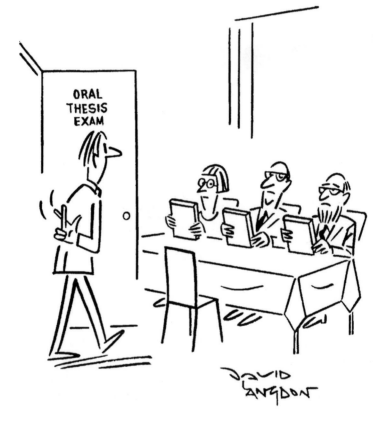

Viva

Submitting a thesis and preparing for the *viva voce* examination

As the time for thesis submission approaches, you will feel greatly pressed for time, not least because of the preparations you will be making for your next career move, as well as with trying to get some of your work published. You must resist the urge to be impulsive and remain fastidious in these final stages, particularly when it comes to printing and binding your thesis. In this way, the consternation of noticing that thesis pages are missing, or figures are upside down or mis-labelled in the final bound version can be avoided!

Number of copies

The number of copies you decide to print and bind must take into account how many copies the university requires for submission, and how many it will eventually keep. Some people choose only to print the minimum number required by the university initially and then to print additional copies once any necessary corrections have been made. A sample calculation of the total number is:

University	3 (2 returned)
Personal	1
Supervisor	1
Department	1
Family	1
Total	5

Timing

The printing and binding of your thesis often takes a much shorter time than you expect; usually a week, but it can even be done over two or three days. Nevertheless, it is important to locate the appropriate printer and binder, and find out times and prices, so that you may plan for them.

Printing

Read through your final draft carefully and, if possible, have another person check the draft for errors. Once you have checked and double-checked your thesis, you can choose either to send it to a professional printer or to print it yourself. If you take the latter option, print it out on a high-quality printer. Even if you are well practised with this printer, there will be unacceptable 'bugs' in the data transmission, and errors in the printing. Plan and be ready for them. Having a spare printer cartridge or toner available is advisable, particularly if you anticipate printing outside normal office hours.

Binding

The binding process will vary from place to place and it is important to check the university regulations. Many places offer thesis binding and there are an increasing number of online services. As well as choosing the colour of the cover, you need to decide whether to have your thesis hard bound or soft bound. Hard-bound theses look more professional and are often required for the final version submitted to the university, but are more expensive. Soft-bound theses can be either bound with cloth spine or with a plastic comb spine. The former is the most popular choice for initial submission as it still looks professional but is cheaper than hard bound. Remember, though, that it is not possible to re-bind the pages from a thesis, so any corrections you make will require a complete new print out.

Submitting

Congratulations! You have now reached the penultimate hurdle. Treasure your beautifully prepared volumes and package and submit them to your university in exactly the fashion it requires.

Preparing for the *viva voce*

Most candidates for a higher degree by thesis will have an oral examination. Consult your university regulations to find out whether this is obligatory, customary, unusual or never occurs for your particular degree. Some oral examinations include the supervisor, but in most cases you will only encounter two or three independent examiners.

This is undoubtedly a daunting experience for you; it forms one of the most important days of your professional life and, we can tell you, one that you will never forget! Remember, this is the one examination that you will take in which *you* set the paper! In the days before your examination, you should read through your own copy of the thesis and revise, once again, at least the key references. Arrive early, bring your own copy of your thesis with you and, it should go without saying, turn up neat and tidy. Dirty fingernails can be very off-putting even to the kindest and most considerate examiner.

Usually each examiner in turn asks you questions, and with your replies there may then be subsidiary questions to follow. You are likely to be taken progressively through your thesis, often beginning with a request to provide a summing up of its objectives, contents and significance. You may first be asked some background questions: where are you working now, what are your future plans, what made you take up this particular field of work? The examiners may then probe your knowledge of the literature (and may well allude to their own work in your field), your findings, your conclusions, where you think you have advanced knowledge in your subject, and finally, where future progress may lie.

Remember one most important thing which should comfort you during your ordeal: you probably know, at this particular moment, just as much, if not more, about your area of work as the examiners do. After all, they did not go through all the references over the previous fortnight, nor have they spent the last year or more devoting all their working time to this particular topic!

The usual formal procedure is for you to be dismissed at the end of the examination and for the examiners then to make their recommendation to the university. You should hear your official result in a few days. Many examiners, however, will give you a broad hint of how you fared at the end of your viva along with details of any corrections or additions they feel are required.

Summary
- The day of your *viva voce* examination will probably be one of the most important and memorable days of your professional life.
- Make sure you read through your thesis and key references beforehand.
- Remember, *you* have set the subject of the examination.
- And remember that *you*, at this moment, are likely to know as much, if not more, about the subject than your examiners!

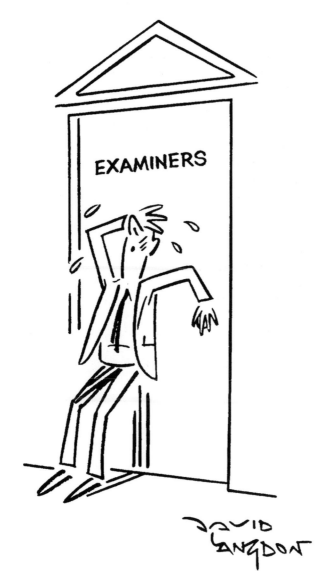

'Phew!'

Further reading

Booth, V. (1993). *Communicating in Science: Writing a Scientific Paper and Speaking at Scientific Meetings*. 2nd edn. Cambridge: Cambridge University Press.

Bradbury, A. (2006). *Successful Presentation Skills*. 3rd edn. London: Kogan Page Ltd.

Goodman, N. W., Edwards, M. B. (2006). *Medical Writing: A Prescription for Clarity*. 3rd edn. Cambridge: Cambridge University Press.

Greenhalgh, T. (2006). *How to Read a Paper: The Basics of Evidence-based Medicine*. Oxford: Wiley-Blackwell.

Gustavii, B. (2003). *How to Write and Illustrate a Scientific Paper*. Cambridge: Cambridge University Press.

Hall, G. (2008). *How to Write a Paper*. 4th edn. Oxford: Wiley-Blackwell.

Kirkman, J. (2005). *Good Style: Writing for Science and Technology*. 2nd edn. Oxford: Routledge.

Medawar, P. B. (1981). *Advice to a Young Scientist*. New York: Basic Books.

Shephard, K. (2005). *Presenting at Conferences, Seminars and Meetings*. London: Sage Publications.

Smith, T. (1999). *Ethics in Medical Research: A Handbook of Good Practice*. Cambridge: Cambridge University Press.

Wang, D., Bakhai, A. (2005). *Clinical Trials: A Practical Guide to Design, Analysis, and Reporting*. London: Remedica.

Appendix: Information for research students wishing to study overseas

International

International handbook of universities and other institutions of higher education. Guide to universities in 108 other countries outside the Commonwealth, USA, Ireland and South Africa. Edited by H. M. R. Keyes and D.J. Aitken, De Gruyter: Hawthorn, NY.

World list of universities. Guide to 6000 universities in 150 countries. De Gruyter: Hawthorn, NY.

Study abroad. Lists scholarships, assistantships, travel grants, international courses in all fields of study, offered, sponsored or administered by more than 70 international organizations. UNESCO Press: Paris.

The grants register. Lists grants, scholarships, special awards, etc., for anyone requiring further professional or occupational training. Edited by Roland Turner. MacMillan Press: London.

The Commonwealth

Commonwealth universities yearbook. The standard guide to the courses, organization, staff and activities of about 500 university institutions of good standing in 29 countries or regions of the Commonwealth. Published annually by the Association of Commonwealth Universities, John Foster House, 36 Gordon Square, London WC1H 0PF, UK.

Scholarships guide for Commonwealth postgraduate students. Published every two years by the Association of Commonwealth Universities, John Foster House, 36 Gordon Square, London WC1H 0PF, UK.

Awards for Commonwealth university staff. Fellowships, visiting professorships, grants, etc. open to university staff in a commonwealth country wishing to study in another country. Published every two years by the Association of Commonwealth Universities, 36 Gordon Square, London WC1H 0PF, UK.

Awards for postgraduate study overseas. Handbook of grants 1 & 2 (edited by M. Brown). Handy, concise lists of recurring scholarships and grants for postgraduates, post doctorates and academics studying in Australia. For Australians and citizens of other countries. Available from the Graduate Careers Council of Australia, PO Box 28, Parkville, Victoria 3052, Australia or scholarships office of the local University. Free of charge.

Graduate study at universities in Britain. A short student information paper including the names of guides to advanced study or research in separate subjects. Association of Commonwealth Universities, 36 Gordon Square, London WC1H 0PF, UK. (Stamped addressed envelope or two International Reply coupons required.)

British universities guide to graduate study. Published every two years by the Association of Commonwealth Universities, 36 Gordon Square, London WC1H 0PF, UK.

Higher education in the United Kingdom. Published every two years by the Association of Commonwealth Universities, 36 Gordon Square, London WC1H 0PF, UK.

Research strengths of universities in the developing countries of the Commonwealth. A register of what universities in the developing countries can offer in the way of research facilities to staff and graduate students. Published by the Association of Commonwealth Universities, 36 Gordon Square, London WC1H 0PF, UK.

Postgraduate study at universities in Britain. A short informational paper containing the names of guides to advanced study or research in separate subjects. Association of Commonwealth Universities, 36 Gordon Square, London, England WC1H 0PF, UK.

United States of America

American universities and colleges. The standard guide to universities and colleges in the US. Edited by W. Todd Furniss. American Council of Education, 1 Dupont Circle, Washington DC 20036, USA.

A selected list of fellowship opportunities and aids to advanced education for United States citizens and foreign nationals. The Publications Office, National Science Foundation, 1800 G Street, NW, Washington DC 20550, USA.

Graduate programs and admissions manual. Information on postgraduate programmes in the USA. Includes details on the admissions processes, financial aid, test requirements, student–staff ratios and full addresses of all listed institutions. Education Testing Service, Princeton, NJ 08541, USA.

Entering higher education in the United States: a guide for students from other countries. New York, College Board, Publications Orders, Box 2815, Princeton, NJ 08541, USA.

Financial planning for study in the United States. New York, College Board, Publications Orders, Box 2815, Princeton, NJ 08541, USA.

The college handbook. Describes more than 2800 US colleges and universities with basic information about each one. New York, College Board, Publications Orders, Box 2815, Princeton, NJ 08541, USA.

Australian–American Postgraduate Foundation, PO Box 1559, Canberra City, ACT 2601, Australia. This organization provides information on study in the US. They stress that financial aid for US universities and colleges, usually in the form of assistantships and tuition waivers, is difficult to get. Information regarding financial aid can only be obtained from the institutions themselves by writing to the appropriate department head of the financial aids office of the individual institution.

Index